BIOMAGNETIC AND HERBAL THERAPY

Michael Tierra, OMD

LOTUS
PRESS

Twin Lakes, WI 53181

DISCLAIMER

This book is a reference work, not intended to diagnose, prescribe or treat. The information contained herein is in no way to be considered as a substitute for consultation with a licensed health-care professional.

Photographs by Thomas Burke.
Model Shasta Tierra.

First Edition 1997

Printed in the United States of America

ISBN 0-914955-33-0

Library of Congress Catalogue No. 96-80512

CONTENTS

Foreword

5

Introduction

7

Herbs and Biomagnetic Therapy

12

Treatment Protocols for Specific Conditions

61

Appendix

81

FOREWORD

I am very pleased to have the opportunity to write a few words about the most recent work of Dr. Michael Tierra in the field of alternative healing. Dr. Tierra has been a pioneer in the field for nearly thirty years, and is always willing to look at the methods used by others and learn from them. His life work, his mission, has been to bring natural healing modalities to people everywhere. As his publisher, it has been my pleasure to read and learn from his research.

I am especially intrigued by his Biomagnetic and Herbal Therapy because of a unique personal insight I gained during a visit to a teaching hospital in South India. That experience gave me the foundation to appreciate what Dr. Tierra has accomplished here.

I met a research scientist at the Jipmer Hospital, Pondicherry, India about 10 years ago. He was doing research on Kirlian photography. Kirlian photography is also known as "aura photography". In essence, it is able to show the bio-magnetic/electric field around any being. He showed me hundreds of such photographs of subjects that had varying levels of radiating energy, depending on their state of mind and their state of health. He took photographs of my hand and then had me undertake some prayers and focused concentration and showed me how these efforts dramatically enhanced the energy field.

Of quite remarkable interest was the series of experiments he had conducted on mice. While I personally am not a supporter of animal testing, I nevertheless was willing to see the results of the work he had been doing for a number of years. He indicated that he had implanted cancerous tumours into a number of mice and over the period of a month had done a series of Kirlian photographs beginning with the healthy (pre-implantation) mice, and monitored the progression of the mice as the tumours developed and affected their health. The difference in the energy field was dramatic.

Of even more consequence, however, was the second stage of his experiments. He had a radionic energy generator that he tuned to the frequency of the healthy mice. He then projected the healthy frequency back onto the tumour-infected mice. The Kirlian photographs showed a remarkable progression of the mice returning to absolute, 100% health, their tumours growing successively smaller and eventually disappearing under this bio-energetic treatment using only the electro-magnetic spectrum as a modality.

I was reminded of this scientist when I read Dr. Tierra's book for the first time, and I realized that here was a practical application of the principles of subtle energetics that were demonstrated by the researcher in India. In this book, Dr. Tierra shows how it is possible for each of us to dramatically affect our bio-magnetic energy. This is done by polarising, directing, and moving our life energy to promote healing and health for each one of us.

The paradigm of health in the future is based on energy flow. This paradigm reaches back to the ancient healing arts of the traditional Chinese, the Ayurvedic and the Native American cultures. It is connected to the work of Hippocrates in ancient Greek culture, and found its way through the herbal and homeopathic science that has flourished in Europe over the last few hundred years.

If we recognize the truths that underlie all these systems, we see that there is a bio-magnetic energy that fills and informs our lives and our bodies, that creates health when it is flowing normally, or disease when it is blocked or hindered in its motion.

Dr. Tierra has advanced this paradigm another step by giving us a practical, insightful and experience-based look at the use of magnets as healing agents.

Santosh Krinsky
President
Lotus Press
Twin Lakes, Wisconsin

INTRODUCTION

Magnetic energy is the structural force of the universe. As such, it is the order that allows the stars and planets throughout the galaxies to revolve and spin at incredible velocities while remaining in their respective orbits. As one of the four fundamental forces of nature, along with gravity, nuclear energy and radioactivity, electromagnetism is related to the Traditional Chinese Medicine (TCM) concept of 'Qi,' the East Indian Ayurvedic definition of 'Prana,' as well as the Hawaiian concept of 'Manas'. These concepts are what many in the West regard as the 'life force'.

Personally, I have had many occasions to experiment with and use magnets, beginning with myself and then extending to family, friends, students and patients. Two particular occasions on myself were most convincing. Both were soft tissue injuries — one to my elbow and the other a ligament injury of my knee which I will describe later.

The elbow pain originated from an unknown cause, perhaps an injury or strain. It had persisted for at least two weeks; during that time I tried acupuncture and herbal treatments which offered only minor temporary relief. As is well known, soft tissue injuries can take some time for repair. It would be most helpful, however, if there was a simple, non-invasive method to hasten the healing and relieve the pain during that time.

I decided to experiment with magnets to treat the problem. While I had previously heard of magnet therapy, I had no personal experience or further knowledge of their use. When I taped a small 1000 Gauss acuband magnet directly on the skin over the 'trigger' point or center of the pain in my arm, I was amazed to find that the pain almost completely disappeared within 5 minutes. I decided to experiment further, first by removing and reapplying the magnet a few times. Each time, the pain returned when the magnet was removed and all but completely disappeared again when reapplied. I then experimented by turning the magnet over to change its polarity from North, which is cooling and dispersing, to South, which is heating and building. I discovered that when the South side of the magnet was against the skin the pain intensified, and by reversing the magnet to North it was alleviated.

Since that time, I have been intrigued with the therapeutic possibilities of bio-magnetic therapy. However, I still had no idea whether the magnet treatment to my arm was only symptomatic or could eventually promote complete healing. Further, I found that there was discrepancies both in print and from various distributors concerning the importance and definition of the North and South sides of a magnet. Despite my confusion, I tentatively began to use magnets on my patients. Because, however, I had such an unsure grasp of any basic theoretical or practical methodology, my results were inconclusive.

I say all this because there may be others who feel unsure about the value and results of an experience with biomagnetic therapy. Through my example, they may appreciate confirmation by someone who has become fully convinced that biomagnetic therapy may well be one of the safest and most powerful natural healing methods ever discovered by humankind, especially for the relief of pain and inflammation.

My interest in magnets was rekindled a few years later when I had a crippling soft tissue injury to the medial aspect of my right knee. It was particularly debilitating because there were few positions either standing, sitting or reclining that could provide relief. Having nearly all but forgotten about my previous experience with the magnets on my elbow, I began by using acupuncture, Moxibustion (heat applied to specific acupuncture points) and herbal poultices, fomentations and liniments. Everything helped, but I still could barely walk or find a comfortable position to either sit or recline.

I certainly was not looking forward to having to stand all day at a forthcoming natural products trade show that included a promised diversion to my excited young son to a nearby entertainment park. In desperation I remembered the all-but-forgotten magnets that I stored in a cupboard near my bed. I systematically applied the North magnets to the trigger points located near the site of pain around my knee. Estimating what meridians were involved, I positioned the South magnets further up the femur and hip on the Gall Bladder and Bladder Meridians. I found, however, that it was the local application of the North magnets around the knee that was most effective. Within two hours after their application, the pain was 95% gone.

Again, I decided to conduct the same experiments on my knee that I had done a few years previous on my elbow pain. By removing and reapplying them, changing the magnets to irrelevant locations and reversing their polarity to South seeking, the pain intensified and my previous findings were absolutely corroborated. I eventually discovered that I needed to wear the magnets on the trigger points around my knee nearly continuously for about two months before the problem became sufficiently stabilized and resolved.

After this second powerful experience with bio-magnetic therapy, I decided to apply magnets on all my patients along with the acupuncture, dietary and herbal therapy that was part of my normal practice. I wanted to discover for myself the range of their effectiveness for a wide variety of complaints. Since that time, I have found biomagnetic therapy to be approximately 90% effective for the relief of pains and conditions caused by inflammation. For example, a woman diagnosed with colitis had tried many forms of conventional and non-conventional treatment over the previous year, but was relieved with the application of magnets to her lower abdomen within a week. Another man with arthritis in his hands and fingers with only minimal response from acupuncture and herbal therapy used magnetic balls to relieve and eventually remedy his condition completely. Similarly, another man had encroaching stiffness in his fingers that was threatening to impair his main preoccupation, the guitar. He also found the results he was seeking with the use of magnetic balls. As a pianist, I can only imagine the benefit these simple magnetic balls could be to the many who have suffered repetitive injury.

Everyone who had acute or chronic lower back, elbow or knee problems found relief, and in many cases complete recovery was achieved from the local application of magnets. Patients with asthma found that the application of magnets to their upper back or chest would provide them the relief they desperately needed without any further external medication. The list goes on to include patients with upper respiratory allergies, gastro-intestinal and digestive complaints, migraine headaches — all were relieved with the use of magnets — and the list of conditions continues to expand. Now with the expanded methods of application using magnetized water, magnetized oils, magnetic mattresses and mattress pads, jewelry and so forth, I am convinced that there is no condition for which bio-magnetic therapy would not be at least helpful.

Because of my experience with traditional Eastern systems of medicine, including Traditional Chinese Medicine (TCM) and East Indian Ayurvedic medicine, I was able to tangibly experience the fundamental energetic basis of healing with magnets described in various traditional healing systems around the world.

I could tangibly understand that the North seeking side of a magnet was equivalent in energy to the definition in TCM of Yin, or in Ayurveda, of Shakti energy. The South facing side was equivalent to TCM Yang, or Ayurvedic Shiva energy. I also understood that the relative strength of a magnet determined whether it was to be used as an important energetic nutrient when in low strength (under 1000 gauss), or a high powered therapeutic tool in high strength (over 3000 gauss). Like other forms of natural healing energy, if reasonably used, magnets are very forgiving. Except for the obvious contraindications noted in the text, it is rare that anyone would experience anything more than a minor discomfort or aggravation, usually caused by using magnets that are too strong, applying the wrong North-South polarity for a given area or generally an overexposure to a strong magnetic field. If, for instance, one misapplies them over a wrong area, uses the wrong polarity or uses magnets that are too strong, there may be a period of minor aggravation and discomfort that is easily remedied as soon as their polarity is reversed or removed. As with herbs, acupuncture and all other systems of natural healing, trial and error is a valid approach to biomagnetic therapy. Here it is importnat to recognize the difference between the harmful, deranging effects of electromagnetic energy which is alternating or AC current, as opposed to the more organizing direct current (DC), energy of permanent magnets.

Science recognizes a close relationship between electricity and magnetism. In 1820, Hans Oersted of Denmark discovered a direct relationship between electricity and magnetism by showing that an electric current flowing in a wire caused a nearby compass needle to be deflected. Following the discoveries of Oersted, Ampere, the 18th century physicist whose notable achievements were germinal to the harnessing of electrical energy, discovered a quantitative relationship between the strength of an electric current and the magnetic field it creates (Ampere's theorem). Noting the close relationship between electricity and magnetism, he described magnetism as "electricity thrown into curves." To reiterate, health represents a balance of positive and negative forces described in TCM as Yin and Yang, in Ayurvedic medicine as 'Shiva' and 'Shakti', and in Western physiology as the sympathetic and parasympathetic systems. Magnets, with their North and South polarity, rerpresent a graphic representation of that universal bipolar energy.

The current theory of free radicals as the cause of degenerative diseases and aging is based on the concept of a negatively charged electron spinning out of its orbit, invading another cell which in turn causes a cellular disruption that sends other subatomic particles off their respective orbits. This results in cellular chaos. Biomagnetic healing is able to passively provide a stimulus for the restoration of balance at a subatomic level and offset the devastating domino-effect of harmful free radicals.

Because every atom generates an electromagnetic (EM) field, we, along with all of nature, are imbued with the power of electromagnetism. It is also possible for us to channel our innate positive electromagnetic energy for healing both ourselves and others.

HERBS AND BIOMAGNETIC THERAPY

The traditional understanding of herbal medicine extends far beyond the mere classification of the biochemical constituents of plants. Imbued with their own unique cellular subatomic electromagnetism, plants are capable of carrying a positive and negative charge. These are appropriately described in traditional herbalism as 'heating' or 'cooling' energies and correspond to their therapeutic properties and flavors and more ambiguously to their various shapes, textures and colors.

Herbs that are eliminative such as chickweed, mint, malva leaf, plantain, and red clover Echinacea, or laxative herbs such as rhubarb root and cascara are understood to be cooling and would have a negative polarity; those that are warming and stimulating such as ginger, cayenne, cloves, angelica or ginseng would have a warming or positive polarity. Stressing the importance of electromagnetism, Einstein said, "We may therefore regard matter as being constituted by the regions of space in which the field is extremely intense . . . .There is no place in this new kind of physics both for the field and matter, for the *field is the only reality* ." (Our italics) From this we see how it is not so much the intrinsic nutritional components of herbs that are responsible for their healing energies, but the stimulating effects corresponding to Einstein's "field" that triggers the healing response. The mystic founder of Theosophy, Madame Blavatsky, states a similar idea in different terms when she describes: "Matter is spirit at its lowest level and spirit is matter at its highest level."

It is said that what may be described as matter, the nucleus of an atom, is so infinitesimal that if we were to gather all the nuclei of a human body, it would be no larger than a period at the end of a sentence. Thus, modern physics theorizes that what we call matter may not be particles at all, but the presence of an impenetrable electro-magnetic field. Life, comprised of a complex chain of bio-chemical and physiological processes is activated and animated by an invisible bio-magnetic force such it finds expression in the food we eat and the herbs we use for medicine. In this regard, Dr. F.K. Bellokossy of Denver, Colorado described life as an "infinitely intelligent interaction of electro-magnetic energies carried by chemical substances."

Modern medicine has come to depend upon such high tech diagnostic procedures as the electro-cardiogram (ECG), the electroencephalogram (EEG), and the electromyogram (EMG) to measure the electrical activity in the heart, the cerebral cortex and the skeletal muscles respectively. If there were no electrical energy in the body, such tests would not be possible.

From the perspective of bio-magnetics, health is based upon the individual cells of the body vibrating at a characteristic normal frequency. Disease, on the other hand, represents an abnormal change in cellular vibration. The therapeutic application of magnets and herbs, at the deepest level, is based on the principle of restoring normal cellular vibration.

This understanding should make magnetic therapy very accessible to those who have an energetic approach to treatment, and it would include traditional herbalism, TCM, Ayurveda and some Western 'holistically' oriented mind-body therapies.

MAGNETIC FORCE: A FUNDAMENTAL EARTH NUTRIENT

The Earth's magnetic field strength is about a half gauss.[1] While seemingly small, the magnetic field strength of gauss as a measure is in proportion to the total mass of the magnet. With that, a half gauss in proportion to the size of the Earth becomes very significant. As a matter of fact, it is essential to life.

With the exploration of space in the 1960's, there came increased awareness of the importance of magnetism in maintaining health. It was found that astronauts, beyond the protective magnetic field of the Earth, often returned with symptoms of psychiatric disturbances, calcium and mineral deficiencies, and other physiological disturbances. Conversely, companies who needed to conduct experiments or manufacture biological products outside of the magnetic field of the earth were, and continue to be, major investors in the space program. Since that time, an integral aspect of space flight research involves studying the effects of magnetic fields on living organisms in space travel.

Part of the Earth's magnetic field is created by the 'ionosphere'— a layer of air containing electrically-charged particles that extend from sixty to one hundred miles above the surface of the Earth. Extending some thousands of miles into space is the 'magnetosphere', sometimes called the Van Allen Belt, after the scientist who discovered it. This is a huge swarm of particles that are threatening to life due to their radioactivity. If it were not for the fact that the harmful particles are trapped by the Earth's magnetic field, life on Earth would be impossible.

The half gauss strength of the Earth seems to be in a state of cyclic change, so that over time the Earth's magnetic poles have repeatedly shifted and changed their location. Scientific research estimates that these reversals occur approximately every half to one million years. The most recent reversal occurred about 700,000 years ago. It has been documented that the Earth's magnetic field has diminished about 50% of what it was 500-1000 years ago, with a full 5% decline recorded in the last 100 years. Drs. Barnwell and Brown of the Department of Biological Sciences, Northwestern University, USA, conducted a number of experiments exposing living organisms to magnetic fields and reported that, "There remains no reasonable doubt that all living organisms are extraordinarily sensitive to magnetic fields." Research on the effect of magnetic fields on living organisms continues in the USA and throughout the world, but some of the most important research is that done by the Japanese. From this we can appreciate the vital importance of geomagnetic energy to life.

MAGNETIC FIELD DEFICIENCY SYNDROME

Dr. Kyoichi Nakagawa, MD, Director of Isuzu hospital, Tokyo, Japan, has described a pathological condition called Magnetic Field Deficiency Syndrome (MFDS) [2] that causes a variety of symptoms including stiff shoulders, back and neck, chest pains, habitual constipation and general fatigue.

He mailed questionnaires to 11,648 Japanese users of magnets 2.5 mm thick x 5 mm in diameter with external gauss strength of 590. Only the North magnetic side was in direct contact with the skin for treatment in these studies. Women represented 57% and men 43% of the total with a representative age group between 40 and 49 years.

Magnets were used for the following conditions:

Stiff neck and shoulders	45.20%
Lumbago	19.00%

Neuralgia	13.90%
Painful muscles	12.30%
Rheumatism	1.30%
Other	6.30%
No reply	2.00%

Effects were usually noticed from the second to the fourth day. No adverse effects were reported, while over 90% of the users classified results as very efficacious, efficacious or fairly efficacious, and 10% as ineffective or not very effective.

A number of other studies were conducted with 400 subjects in 1976 by professors Akio Yamada and Shuwichi-Hirose of the Faculty of Medicine, University of Tokyo; professor Yamada, University of Juntendo, Tokyo; and Kyoshi Kurmskima, Kohnodai National hospital. Some tests were double-blind placebo using a variety of different magnetic devices. Symptoms addressed included pains in the back of the neck, shoulders, back, arms, hands and legs. Effectiveness was in the range of 60 to 80% within a period of 7 to 14 days. No side effects were reported.

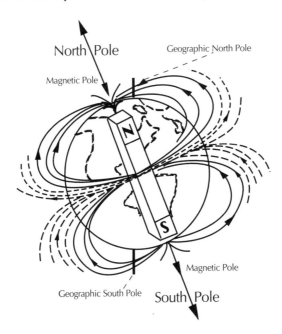

A double-blind study was conducted by Dr. Yoshio Oay treating 80 subjects with lumbar pain using strong magnetic belts containing magnets of 1,500 gauss. Fifty subjects were given the magnetic belts while 30 received placebos or less powerful belts of 200 gauss. All subjects using the full strength belts evidenced marked improvement while those using weaker magnets or placebos showed only slight or no marked improvement.

Some confuse the electro-magnetic energy generated by power lines, computer and TV monitors, electrical wiring in our homes and vehicles as equivalent. These, however, represent alternating current (AC) which is deranging to normal cellular metabolism. The earth and other metallic substances, in contrast, represent a permanent magnetic field or direct current (DC) which can be integrative to the sub-atomic particles of cells.

Many factors, beside the natural cyclic waxing and waning of geomagnetic activity, contribute to the diminishing of direct current (DC) magnetic energy to our body. Some of these are the result of interference from the AC current of man-made electromagnetic radiation which is incompatible with our bodies' biomagnetic emanations; these include television, radio, radar, household appliances, computers, electrical wiring in buildings, nearby power lines and other sources.

The effects of working and living in concrete and steel structures further cut us off from the Earth's direct magnetic force. The automobile, train, jet plane, bus and other hi-tech modes of travel are other ways we are deprived of important natural magnetism from the Earth. Shrinking open spaces, living high above sea level on ground covered with concrete and asphalt and the decreasing amount of ground water all contribute to lack of conductivity and Magnetic Field Deficiency Syndrome (MFDS).

The magnetic field of our planet is responsible for the natural biorhythms of life. In Traditional Chinese Medicine these biorhythms describe how Qi or bio-magnetic force is concentrated in certain areas of the body according to cycles of each day and season. It may also be concentrated in certain areas on the Earth that inexplicably have been able to retain their magnetic strength. There are recognized earth healing areas such as Lourdes, France and Sedona, Arizona.

Symptoms of MFDS may be similar to a variety of chronic conditions such as chronic fatigue syndrome, candida albicans and environmental allergies. MFDS typically is associated with a general malaise and low energy, frequent susceptibility to disease, tightness of the neck and shoulders, fibro-myalgic body pains, forgetfulness, headaches, digestive and circulatory problems and a general 'foggy' feeling.

At many healing retreats that I have both attended and conducted, we would hug a tree to experience the grounding of accumulated unnatural magnetic distortions. While this may be impossible to scientifically prove, anecdotally everyone who has ever hugged a tree will acknowledge a certain feeling of well-being afterwards, characterized by a lessening of mental and physical heaviness. Perhaps, this is another indication of an innate need for a certain type of natural energy that is lacking in our daily lives.

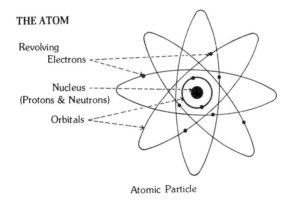

THE ATOM

Revolving Electrons

Nucleus
(Protons & Neutrons)

Orbitals

Atomic Particle

HOW DO MAGNETS WORK?

Magnetic forces have such all-encompassing, powerful effects that no one description of how they exert their positive therapeutic effects could adequately describe all the many complex ways they affect mind and body. However, one theory, based on the concept of diseased cells losing their magnetic equilibrium, explains how topically applied magnets are able to support and encourage the normal functional relationship both within the molecular structure of each cell as well as positively influencing the relationships throughout the entire body-mind process.

Another theory is that magnets exert a powerful attraction to the iron content in the blood, penetrating the outer layers of skin, muscle and fatty tissue to the capillaries that feed directly into the bloodstream. By attracting iron and perhaps other inorganic molecules to a diseased area, circulation is increased. This is enhanced by the increase of oxygen and other vital nutrients to the affected site that assists in healing. The combined effect is regulating the pH of the cells and tissues, balancing, ionizing and oxygenating them and generally relieving congestion and pain by improving blood circulation.

Scientific research documents the following specific physiological effects of biomagnetic therapy:[3]

1. It effects increased blood and oxygen circulation along with the nutrient carrying potential of the blood.

2. It is able to affect pH balance (acid-alkaline) which is often imbalanced in diseased tissues.

3. It positively speeds up the migration of calcium ions to facilitate the healing of nervous tissue and bones (usually in at least half the time). Because of this it can also help remove the pathological buildup of calcium associated with arthritic joints.

4. It can powerfully influence the production of certain hormones from the various endocrine glands.

5. It stimulates and fosters enzyme activity and other related physiological processes.

If we consider that all functions of the body are essentially biomagnetic, we can understand how each body cell, down to the DNA, has a positive and negative biomagnetic field and that cell division is fundamentally a magnetic process that occurs throughout the various tissues and organs of the body. Physiological biochemistry that utilizes various amino acids appears to be helped by biomagnetism. It has been found that the pineal gland, a tiny pine-cone shaped gland located directly in the center of the brain, is responsible for the production of melatonin, enzymes, immune function, oxidation, carbohydrate metabolism, pigmentation by melanin and the cyclic patterns of sleep and awakening. It is regulated, according to Robert Becker in his book on biomagnetics called *Cross Currents*, "by exposure to steady magnetic fields of the same strength as the geomagnetic field". Since the pineal gland

and melatonin govern stress tolerance and the production of antioxidants that help control the harmful effects of free radicals that cause degenerative disease and aging, biomagnetic therapy can have a very beneficial effect in helping to regulate the pineal gland; this offsets the unnatural disruption of our exposure to artificial geo-magnetic fields.

The following chart derived from Bengallineville's book, *Magnet Therapy: Theory and Practice*, outlines the various factors that are responsible for cellular magnetic disturbances:

Extrinsic Factors		Intrinsic Factors
Natural	*Artificial*	
		Emotional stress
Solar flares	X-rays	Hormonal imbalances
Sunspot activity	Cobalt-60	Infectious or pathogenic microorganisms
Eclipses	Radium implants	Deficiencies (iodine deficiency produces thyroid imbalances)
Moon phases (new and full moon)	Nuclear plants using radioactive substances like Strontium-90 and Plutonium	Deficient or imbalanced diet
Thunderstorms	Radiation from color televisions and computer monitors	Ovulation
Cosmic rays	Radiation from microwave ovens	Injuries (serious)
X-rays	Chemical additives in food	Injurious habits like excessive intake of alcohol and drugs
Subsoil radiation (geopathic zones)	Radioactive fallout from nuclear tests	Pregnancy
Certain planetary confugurations	Irradiated wheat and other foods	Menopausal period
	High tension cables	
	Sound vibrations	
	Aluminum vessels used in cooking	

THE SAFETY OF BIOMAGNETIC THERAPY

According to my personal experience and the experience of biomagnetic therapists and patients from around the world, magnets are corrective and regulating and therefore have little risk of either dependency or negative interaction with drugs. Magnets under 2500 gauss seem to be safe regardless of their North - South polarity. Nevertheless, as a kind of energetic nutrient when used or worn daily in a mattress or shoe insole, I prefer using magnets no stronger that 1000 gauss strength. Over 3000 gauss strength, prolonged exposure to the wrong magnetic field polarity can create a minor imbalance in a small percentage of people. Therefore, exposure to high strength magnetic fields should be limited to a period of no longer than 30 minutes at a time, once or twice daily. This is generally not true, however, of small high-powered acuband magnets which can be left on the affected site for days, provided the correct North-South magnetic field is in use.

I once met a woman who was treating herself for a year for candida albicans and attendant symptoms, using very high strength magnets on a daily basis. She became frightened when she discovered that her hair began to fall out. This occurred, despite the fact that most of her other symptoms were alleviated, and she even claimed to feel more energetic and vital than ever. Because the thought of losing her hair was so frightening to her, she resolved never to get near a magnet again. One day I was gratefully surprised to find a varied collection of high grade industrial strength magnets deposited in the waiting room of my clinic. I later asked her what she felt about the use of magnetic mattresses. She asserted that there was no comparison with her unfortunate experience and that their relatively low gauss strength made them virtually impossible to cause any significant harmful reaction.

Given the fact that it is impossible to predict what is otherwise known as an idiosyncratic reaction that an individual may have to practically any substance or thing, overwhelmingly the potential benefits of biomagnetic therapy makes it well worth a try for a wide variety of conditions.

THE TREATMENT OF CANCER WITH MAGNETS

For serious diseases such as cancer, it is best to combine a variety of therapeutic approaches — dietary, herbal, nutritional supplements — along with the local application of magnets over the affected site. Based on the findings and studies of Drs. Davis, Wollin and Philpott, the local application of magnets over tumors has in many instances proven to be effective in bringing about a remission or diminishing of their size, or at least lessening or controlling pain without the use of drugs.

Dr. Philpott's book[4] is extremely informative and highly convincing, if for no other reason than that it is responsibly cautious in making extravagant claims. He sites a number of valid protocols for treatment and various successful cases where these have been successfully applied.

In terms of treatment, the strongest neodymium magnets are preferred. These should be applied over all sites where there are tumors and should be large enough to cover the entire mass. Because South promotes growth and proliferation and North disperses and inhibits, only the negative magnetic field or bio-north magnet energy should be applied over known tumor or cancer sites. For optimal results the bio-north magnets should be left on continuously. Following Dr. Davis and Wollin's suggestions, bio-south is applied over the thymus gland situated approximately on the sternum between the breasts for 30 minutes each day to stimulate the immune system.

Topically applied magnets are especially effective for malignant skin melanomas. However, they may be useful for all other cancers as well. Dr. Philpott gives various case studies of the treatment of malignant melanomas, as well as a case of prostate cancer.

Dr. Philpott asserts that all cancer tissue is acidic and does not need oxygen to produce ATP (adenosine triphosphate), the basic building block for cellular energy. He postulates that cancer cells produce their own ATP from a "fermentation process and not by oxidative phosphorylation." The acidic state associated with cancer is produced by "many substances such as reactions to foods, chemicals, inhalants including the known carcinogens" which create mutated cancer cells as a result of injured DNA genetic material. These mutated cancer cells clone or reproduce themselves into larger and larger colonies with their own vascularized food supply to form ever enlarging tumors, which in turn break off and spread throughout the body.

Exposing cancer cells to a negative (north) magnetic field seems to have many powerful effects in destroying and/or inhibiting their growth. Again, never apply a South magnet over the site of an active tumor or cancer because it will increase their size and proliferation.

First by normalizing pH, the bio-north facing magnets are able to chemically alter the medium necessary for cancer cells to thrive. The area is therefore permeated with molecular oxygen released from acids, hydrogen peroxide and free radical oxygen. ATP is optimally produced from oxidative, rather than fermentive phosphorylation. Cell division, protein synthesis and microorganism replication necessary for cancer growth are all impaired when exposed to a prolonged negative field. The food supply to cancer cells is cut off because prolonged exposure to a negative magnetic field constricts vascularization or blood flow within the tumor (called angiogenesis) while having no adverse effect on healthy circulation.

A few positive experiences from my own clinical practice may serve to offset any concerns or negative impressions one may have about magnetic therapy. One was the prolonged use of high gauss magnets to completely eliminate and control the pain of a man diagnosed with incurable liver cancer. Because of the use of strong North facing magnets applied over the site of pain, he was able to spend his last days with a minimum amount of discomfort without the use of morphine or any other deadening pain medication. Two women, one with lung cancer and another with breast cancer, were able to minimize or completely eradicate any attendant pains in a similar way. Finally, a man with a diagnosed brain tumor fastened a strong neodymium magnet on a cap which he wore for half to one hour periods twice each day. He was reexamined after a period of several months and doctors were amazed to find that his tumor had significantly diminished in size. I must add that all these patients were given adjunctive dietary and herbal therapy, which I am sure contributed greatly to their response. Certainly, if for no other purpose than the relief of pain, but also for the powerful tumor inhibiting properties of the north magnet, they should be used at least adjunctively with other modalities for the treatment of chronic diseases such as cancer.

Contraindications

Despite the safety of magnets, there are some contraindications to be aware of. First, do not use magnets during pregnancy, on those who have a history of epilepsy, or those wearing a pacemaker. Strong magnets should be used with care on small infants and children, on the eyes, the brain or over the heart.

Healing Crisis Reaction

Because magnets have such a positive effect on vascular circulation, some individuals may experience a temporary aggravation as a consequence of the increased discharge of toxins. Some healing crisis reactions may include symptoms such as light headedness, itching, allergic reaction, headache, sleepiness or a sensation of heat. When this occurs it is best to gradually ease into their use over a period of time.

MAGNETS

Materials used for magnets are those whose atoms can be permanently or semi-permanently lined up. Of all magnetic materials, an alloy comprised of one-fifth boron and four fifths Neodymium makes the most powerful magnet. Other materials used for magnets are Alnico magnets comprised of an alloy of aluminum, nickel, iron, cobalt and copper. These are about 10 times more powerful than steel magnets and 100 times more powerful than the Earth's magnetic field. Ferrite magnets are comprised of carbonates of barium and iron. They are more powerful and significantly cheaper than alnico magnets but have the disadvantage of being very brittle.

MAGNETIC FIELDS

The magnetic field is the area where magnets exert their force. This is easily determined by holding a compass near the magnet to determine if the strength of the magnet overrides the magnetic force of the poles.

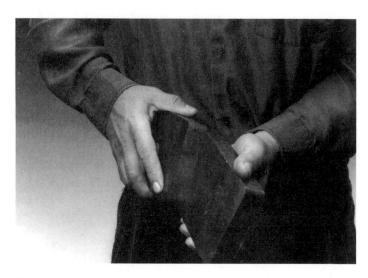

The proper method of handling strong block magnets is to slide them apart or together.

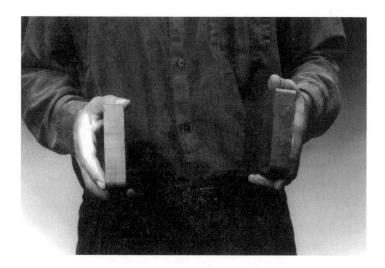

It can be dangerous to allow strong block magnets to slam together. They can injure the fingers or shatter.

MAGNETIC POLES

Up until recently, scientific technical studies of magnets described the nature and effects of the two poles of a magnet as being the same. The years of research by Dr. Albert Roy Davis Ph.D., based on isolating and measuring the effects of the two poles, has confirmed the different reactions they produce on living systems.

Dr. Davis was able to measure the direction of electron spin given off and transmitted from the two ends of magnet's poles. From this, he was able to determine that the spin of the electrons were in reverse of each other. The electrons coming from the South pole of the magnet cycled and moved clockwise, to the right, while those emanating from the North pole moved and cycled to the left, or counterclockwise.[5]

This was confirmed from the use of complex technical magnetometers measuring the magnetic field of Earth from space. It was discovered that magnetic energy moves in a spiral, forming the infinity pattern. Upon leaving either the North or South poles it travels halfway backward, clockwise or counterclockwise depending upon the exiting pole, to reenter and rephase itself inwards, where it takes on the reverse spin in the opposite direction.

Dr. Davis was able to use a cathode ray vacuum to photograph in color the different North and South energies emitted from a long bar magnet. By a series of experiments, first on animals and seeds and then on various fluids and foods, he was able to observe the physical effects on living systems. He confirmed the positive effects of the South pole energies in promoting rapid growth, fertility and a general metabolically heating effect, as opposed to the inhibiting negative effects of the North pole that had a quieting, soothing and metabolically cooling effect.

Using untreated seeds as a comparison guide, Dr. Davis conducted a series of laboratory experiments on seeds and vegetables that were first exposed to the South pole magnet. An analysis of the end products of these plant products showed a noticeable increase in protein, sugars and oils as opposed to the control group. In contrast, those exposed to the North pole were lower in protein, sugars and oils than the control group.

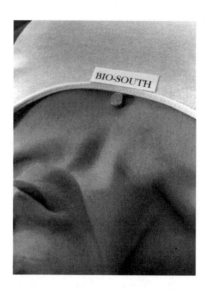

Cancer: South Neodymium magnet over the Thymus gland 30 minutes twice daily to strengthen the immune system.

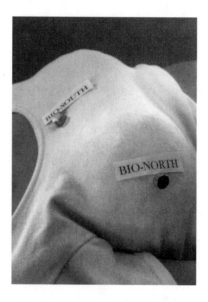

Cancer treatment: North over the tumor site, South over the Thymus. 30 mins twice daily.

He then studied the effect of South and North poles on the development and growth of earthworms. Again, worms treated with South pole energy multiplied faster and grew larger than those treated with North pole energy. The protein of earthworms is approximately 90% on the average, but the effect of the South pole evidenced a marked increase of their protein content. He was also able to corroborate similar results on the growth of mice and rats.

As stated, the difference between magnetized and demagnetized material is that more electrons in a magnetized object are aligned to spin in a single rather than a seemingly randomized direction. The direction follows the magnetic poles of the Earth between the Southern and Northern hemispheres. [6]

Following the system described by Davis and Rawls, the Bio-North (-) pole of a magnet has the same polarity as the true geographic North pole of the Earth. This bio-magnetic definition of North and South is in contradistinction to that of the National Bureau of Standards (NBS).

To determine the North-South direction of a magnet, tie a thread to the center of the magnet bar and the other end to a high place such as a ceiling or door frame. The suspended magnet will tend to spin and eventually position itself in the direction of geographical North and South as is determined by a compass. Perma-

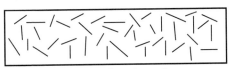

Unmagnetized bar of steel: random electron flow.

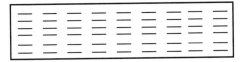

Magnetized bar of steel: organized flow of electrons. Demonstrates the difference between a non-magnetic bar of steel and a magnetic bar.

nently mark as South the side facing the South pole of the magnet with red paint or fingernail polish. With one marked magnet, it can be lined up and used to indicate the polarity of all other magnets.

Another method is to align the needle of a compass to point North. Bring one side or end of the magnet near the compass. The side of the magnet that is able to attract the North end of the compass needle is to be marked as North. All other magnets can be so marked and aligned to conform to one predetermined indicator magnet.

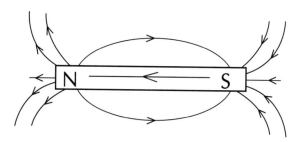

Field of bar magnet. The lines of force emerge from the North pole (N) and converge towards the South pole (S) outside the magnet. Within the magnet the lines of force flow from the South pole to the North pole.

MEASURING THE STRENGTH OF MAGNETS

The power of a magnet is measured in terms of gauss units, with the Earth's surface gauss being approximately 0.5 gauss. The total line of force is called magnetic flux. The gauss or flux density is the line of force per unit area of the pole. Precise gauss measurement is not possible without specially engineered technical instruments. Most commercial magnets are sold and described according to their lifting power. A roughly approximate equivalence of gauss strength to lifting power is as follows:

Lifting Power	Gauss (for larger magnets)
2 pounds	500-600 gauss
5 pounds	900-1200 gauss
25 pounds	2000 gauss
50 pounds	3500-4500 gauss

As can be seen, the lifting power of commercial magnets have a wide range variance. For practical purposes, however, without the purchase of costly measuring instruments, the only way magnet strength can be ensured is to purchase them from manufacturers and reputable distributors (see index).

Magnetic strength is classified as follows:

| Low gauss | 300 - 700 g | High gauss | 3000 - 6000 g |
| Medium gauss | 1000 - 2500 g | Super gauss | 7000 - 12000 g |

The gauss level employed is dependent upon the severity and duration of a complaint, together with the age and condition of the patient. It is always best to begin treatment with a low to medium gauss range and then increase to higher strength as necessary. On infants, young children, the frail and elderly, use only low strength magnets.

Finally, many biomagnetic therapists believe that magnets whose gauss measure less than 2500 can be used irrespective of their North or South polarity. It is my experience that the quickest and most dramatic results occur when the North and South are appropriately applied according to an evaluation of the condition to be treated.

THE CARE AND HANDLING OF MAGNETS

To prevent them from losing their power or becoming broken and destroyed, magnets must be carefully handled. Dropping a magnet or subjecting it to a sharp blow may cause it to lose much of its strength. Furthermore, magnets subjected to temperatures in excess of 500 degrees Fahrenheit will lose all of their energy.

U-shaped magnets need to be placed on a flat bar or cylinder so that both ends of the magnet make contact with the metal. This is called a "Keeper" and prevents the dissipation of their magnetic power. For long, flat, wide surface magnets, bend a piece of iron, a can or a metal bar that can be fastened to both ends to provide a passage of energy between both poles and again prevent its loss into space. Try to keep different sizes and strengths of magnets away from each other to prevent them from bleeding off their charges.

All magnets can be stuck together but they should be positioned so that they are symmetrical in a single row and not balled up in any way with magnets of various sizes hanging off the ends. This is especially true of inferior quality magnets, while with higher quality industrial strength magnets this is not a consideration.

Finally, magnets can be dangerous. The attractive force of two 25 pound magnets is capable of inflicting serious injury by pinching fingers or other bodily parts that may get caught in their way. It is easier to handle strong magnets if they are wrapped in some kind of thin soft fiber such as a cotton towel.

SUMMARY OF PRECAUTIONS IN THE HANDLING AND USE OF MAGNETS

a. Remove battery powered wristwatches and any other magnetic objects whose field can be altered by the presence of an externally applied magnet.

b. Avoid dropping, banging or heating magnets above 500 degrees Fahrenheit as this may dissipate their strength.

c. For U-shaped magnets, use a "keeper" to connect the two ends when it is not in use.

d. Be careful in handling large heavy magnets, as one can injure a body part if they were to suddenly slam together from a distance.

e. If possible, do not allow different sized magnets to remain together.

f. Keep magnets away from homeopathic remedies, computer hard drives, recording tape, credit cards, videos and CD's to prevent their being damaged or erased. Magnets should also be kept away from battery operated watches, hearing aids and from individuals who have a pacemaker or any metallic parts placed in their body.

MAGNET THERAPY

Biomagnetic therapy is used for the control of pain, to stop infections, heal bones and scar tissue, rejuvenation of cells and balancing the body's energy levels. It can also be effectively combined with most other therapeutic modalities. The magnet chosen is based on the strength, shape and size. Some considerations are:

1. duration of the ailment
2. severity of the condition
3. total area to be treated
4. whether the diseased tissue is superficial or deep
5. the patient's sensitivity

Therapeutic Application of the South and North Poles

Understanding and utilizing the unique and sometimes confusing application of the North and South Poles of a magnet is fundamental. The true North side of a magnet is attracted and/or points to the 'true North' polarity of the earth. However, magnet therapy calls the side that is attracted to the 'North polarity' as 'bio-South,' and vice versa. When a magnet attracts the North pointing end of a compass it should be called 'North' or 'bio-North.' The North pole is cooling, sedating and dispersing, corresponding to the traditional Chinese medicine definition of Yin, or negative polarity. The South Polarity is heating, stimulating and accumulating, corresponding to the Yang, or positive polarity.

All descriptions of positive and negative are not qualitative definitions but express the relationship between the opposite poles to each other and outer phenomena.

	Indications	**Contraindications**
SOUTH	Tonifying, strengthening, building, heating, Yang in nature. Can be used for pains caused by weakness, coldness and deficiency (usually of a more chronic and 'achy' nature), also for hypometabolic conditions associated with low energy, weak digestion and weak immune system.	Not for acute inflammatory conditions, bacterial infections, cancers and tumors, excess Yang.
NORTH	Clearing, eliminative, detoxifying, dispersing, cooling, Yin in nature. Can be used for acute pains (sharp or burning) caused by heat, inflammation, hyper-metabolic conditions, hypertensive conditions, insomnia, nervousness, infections and inflammations.	Not for deficiency conditions, coldess, low metabolism, weakness.

SOUTH AND NORTH COMBINED

When pain, infection or another condition has gotten to a point where the body apparently lacks both the positive and negative energies to fully recover, both poles should be applied. This can be done either by alternating the application of North and South every 15 minutes or by applying a number of both North and South acu-magnets simultaneously over an area. This approach can also be used if the site of pain encompasses a large area.

This is equivalent to a deficiency of both Yin and Yang.

This harmonizing approach is one of the most commonly used because conditions are seldom strictly Excess or Deficient. It is especially useful when a single center of the pain or disease extends over a larger area or cannot be discerned. The disadvantage is that if the particular site can be found and appropriately treated, positive results are quicker if the optimum polarity is used.

Therapeutic application of North

The North magnetic pole is inhibiting and sedating. It slows down cellular metabolism. Because of this, it is cooling, soothing and retarding and useful for painful or inflammatory conditions such as: Arthritis, spondylitis, prostatitis, lumbago, chronic and acute headaches, bruises, injuries, sharp pains, bacterial infections, dysentery, skin ailments such as eczema, psoriasis and ringworm, tumors, mental retardation, epilepsy, cataract, glaucoma, neuralgia, nervousness, insomnia and initially on hernias. It can be applied for the initial inflammatory response to any injury. When a condition assumes a more chronic state, however, one may need to switch to the more tonifying South pole to relieve symptoms.

North energies over 7000 gauss retard bacterial growth as well as cell and tissue regeneration. In the September 1990 "Journal of the National Medical Association", it is clearly shown how the North magnetic pole inhibits the growth of lung carcinoma cells. In general, the North polarity tends to have a normalizing effect regardless of the length of exposure.

Therapeutic Application of South

The South magnetic pole is heating, tonifying and augmenting and increases cellular metabolism. It can be used for the following conditions: Paralysis, leucoderma, alopecia, hernia (later), asthma, tingling and numbness, to strengthen weak muscles and tissues, comatose conditions, after debilitating illness such as tuberculosis, gastroenteritis, scars, etc.

Because South promotes growth, it should never be directly applied on cancerous tumors, bacterial or viral infections or parasites. For regeneration of cells and tissues, magnets over 7000 gauss are extremely effective.

Applying Complete North and South Pole Magnetic Therapy

The bioelectrical force of the right side of the body is more Yin and inhibitory. If there is a lack of the Yin-inhibitory force, the left sided Yang-stimulating bioelectrical activity will appear to be in excess. This represents False Yang or Yin Deficiency. It can manifest as apparent hyperactivity with symptoms such as high blood pressure, hyperthyroidism, palpitations, hyperacidity, etc., all within the overall context of Deficiency and wasting. For these conditions, apply a Yang South magnet to the inside of the right wrist to restore equilibrium and harmony.

If the Yang left-sided energies of the body are weaker than the right-sided Yin, there will be hypoactive or apparent excess Yin symptoms. These can include low blood pressure, hypothyroidism, sluggish bowel movements, general lethargy, fluid retention and edema and hypoglycemia. These conditions are treated by applying the South pole to the inside of the left wrist.

Chronic pains, including chronic arthritic and rheumatic pains, may also require bipolar treatment. Treating large organ systems such as the Liver and Kidneys also seems to respond better to the use of bipolar treatment. To speed the mending of fractures, dual poles are used. South should be applied to the upper side of the break and North applied to the lower side. Magnets come in many shapes and forms. The following are some of the more common ones that are used therapeutically.

Bi-polar Magnets and their Therapeutic Applications

In an attempt to utilize the combined North-South poles, various bipolar magnets have been used. In 1981, a Swiss scientist, Arno Latske, introduced an alternating polarity magnet. He observed that when these bipolar magnets were applied over areas of pain, relief and healing occurred; this was due to charged electrolytes in the blood that passed perpendicular to the magnetic field as a result of what is known in physics as the Hall Effect. The North-South poles of the magnet were arranged in perpendicular strips so that the optimal response occurred with blood vessels that directly crossed the bipolar North-South magnetic strips. However, those vessels that did not cross the bipolar arrangement sufficiently had the least therapeutic effect.

Next, a German scientist, Horst Baermann, in an attempt to improve the Hall Effect, developed a magnet with concentric North-South strips. The problem is that if the blood vessels did not cross near the center of the circle, there was little benefit from the alternating current.

In an attempt to circumvent the shortcomings of the previous two designs, an American engineer, Vincent Ardizzone of Nu-Magnetics, Inc., NY, developed a checkerboard design that accommodates the random design of blood vessels. While the previous two designs had only two sides per pole adjacent to opposite poles, the four-sided checkerboard pattern significantly increased the possibility of a blood vessel being exposed to cross alternating poles. This design also allowed for the magnet to be cut into various shapes and sizes without intervening gaps.

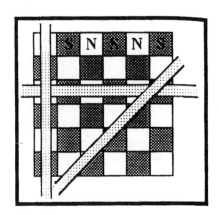

Ardizzone's checkerboard pattern maximizes the therapeutic effect on blood vessels.

Ardizzone's magnets are a patented design exclusive to the Nikken magnetic Wellness products. They are thin and flexible and come in various sizes and shapes for convenient application to various parts of the body. The alternate North and South checkerboard pattern widens the blood vessels to increase blood circulation to the affected area and increase lymphatic flow. By so doing, the body's innate healing processes are increased with the increase of oxygen and vital nutrients and the removal of toxic substances from the compromised tissues.

ACU BAND MAGNETS

These are usually 0.16" dia x 0.06" thick and come with 0.8" dia Band-Aids. They are available in varying gauss strengths and different alloys, usually in packets of 12. The most effective in my experience are acuband magnets that range from 3000 to 9000 gauss. Some are marked with a groove to indicate the North side, while others have a tiny protrusion, indicating the South.

One or more are taped directly over or near the affected site or acupuncture points, using either the North or South polarity as appropriate. Magnets with opposite polarity can be applied directly opposite or distally along a line or acupuncture meridian located nearest the affected area. North or South polarity can be used over acupuncture points and/or centers diagnostically related to the primary symptom.

For instance: For acute colds and flu tape North facing magnets to Large Intestine 4, Large Intestine 11, Triple Warmer 5 and Governor 14. For chronic back ache that is not inflamed, tape South facing magnets over Bladder 23 and Kidney 3. One can apply a North directly over the acute 'trigger' points of pain, and further down the Bladder meridian over Bladder 40 behind the knee.

For insomnia apply a North magnet to Yintang point between the eyebrows and two North magnets to one of the two Anmien points behind the ear.

For fatigue and low energy apply South magnets to Stomach 36, Conception vessel 6 or 4 and Bladder 23 on the lower back. In addition, one can also apply a North magnet to Large intestine 4 on the hand to help clear any Heat and toxicity.

For promoting the healing of fractures apply alternating South and North magnets directly along the affected area. These can be simultaneously used with North to reduce any inflammation in the area.

These are only a few of many possibilities based on a knowledge of acupuncture meridians and points. It is a good idea to have a razor available to shave off any hair that may prevent the Band-Aid from sticking. Acu-magnets can be left on for a week, taken off briefly and reapplied if they are still needed. If there is any prolonged aggravation or discomfort, they should be removed or reverse the North-South polarity.

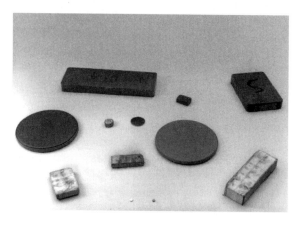

Various shapes and sizes of magnets.

Large Block Magnets

These are iron ferrite magnets which can be purchased from industrial magnet manufacturers and come in various sizes and very high Gauss. Since these are made of fragile ceramic, they are not easy to handle. In general one should learn the technique of sliding them apart or together when needed and keep delicate fingers out of the way in case they inevitably snap together.

Smaller ones can be ordered in various sizes and dimensions and are available in dual color to easily distinguish between the North and South polarity. The strength of these magnets may be

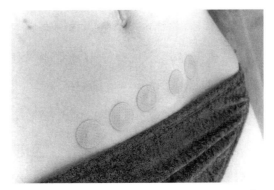

North acuband magnets for colitis, constipation and painful menstruation.

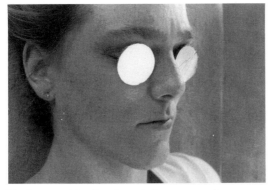

North acuband magnets for cysts and fibroids.

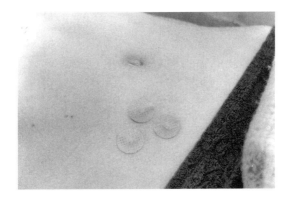

North or combined and south flex magnets for conjunctivitus, injuries, cataracts and glaucoma.

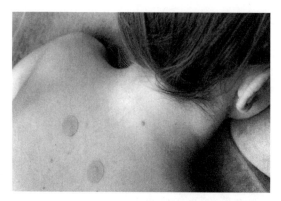

Asthma and lung problems. North acuband magnets
1 1/2" out fom spine between the 2nd and 3rd vertebrae.

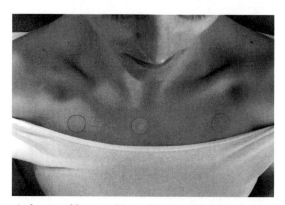

Asthma and lung problems. North acuband magnets
for asthma.

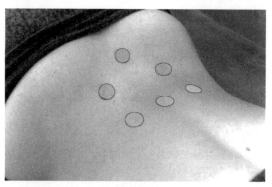

North Acuband magnets for back pain.

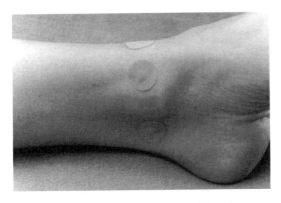

North acuband magnets for treating ankle pain.

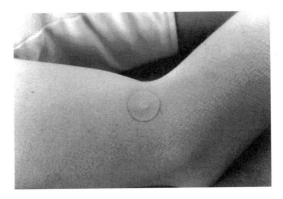

North acuband magnets on large intestine acupoint
for elbow pain and skin disease.

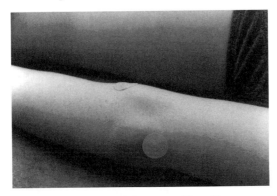

Acuband magnet on triple warmer 10 and large
intestine 11 for elbow pain.

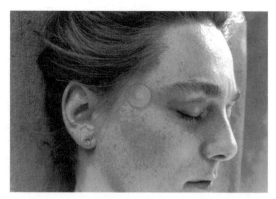

North acuband magnet for treatment of headache.

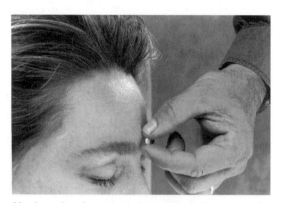

North acuband magnet being applied without tape for headache, nervousness and insomnia.

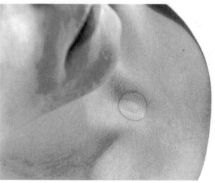

North acuband magnet for cough.

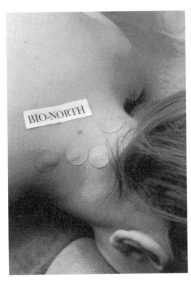

North acuband magnets for neck tightness and pain.

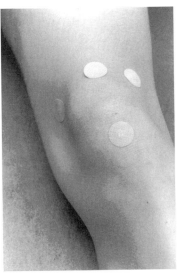

North acuband magnets for knee pain and weakness.

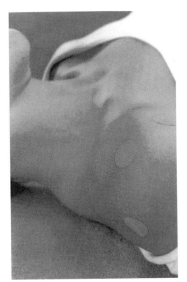

North acuband magnet for treating shoulder pain.

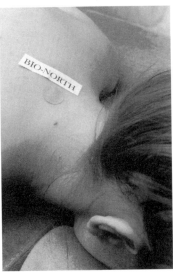

North magnet point for stimulating the immune system- placed on the spine between the 7th cervical and 1st thoracic vertebrae. Also good for treatment and prevention of colds and the flu.

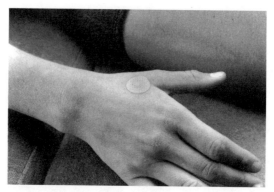

North acuband magnet on large intestine 4 for
diseases of the upper body and inflammatory
diseases.

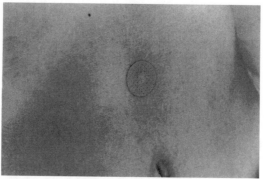

North acuband magnet for stomach pains, indigestion
and nausea. Magnet is placed on center line of
abdomen between navel and base of sternum.

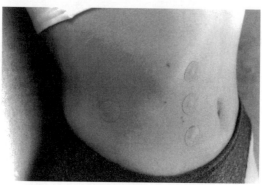

North acuband magnets for liver and gall bladder
diseases.

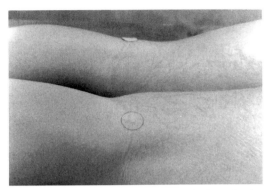

South acuband magnet on Bladder 40 for lower back weakness and pain and disease below the navel.

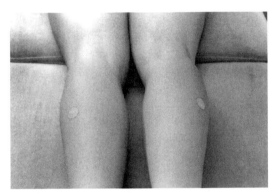

South acuband magnet on Bladder 57 for lower back weakness and pain.

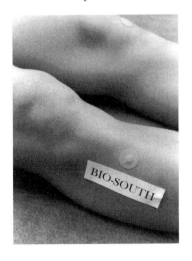

South acuband magnet over energy tonification joint of leg (stomach 36).

deceptive. They are usually available from 1000 to 3600 gauss or higher. Because they cover a larger area, even a lower strength magnet can exert a powerful therapeutic effect. Two magnets can be used to attach to clothing, North or South as needed.

The highest Gauss magnets are Neodymium (NeoMax) magnets. They are composed of iron, boron and neodymium, one of the rarest metals on Earth, and their strength ranges from 2000 to 3600 gauss. Their use was first promoted by the International Medical Research Center based on the discovery and work of Professor Goesta Wollin's development of a Universal Cancer Spiral Theory. Professor Wollin discovered that spirals are found throughout nature, down to the basic shape and structure of DNA. In 1987, the Swedish press widely reported Professor Wollin's discovery of the Universal Cancer Spiral. He claimed that when supermagnets are applied to cancerous tumors, the magnetic spirals, which are larger, would superimpose themselves and destroy the smaller cancerous cell spirals.

Professor Wollin's round neodymium magnets were specifically developed to treat cancer. Usually they are sold in pairs. The North sided magnet is intended to be placed directly over the cancer or tumor while the South is worn over the thymus located on the sternum between the breasts. This is used to help stimulate the body's immune system. While the North magnet directly over the site of the cancer can be left on for a prolonged period, the South over the thymus should only be applied twice daily for no longer than 30 minutes.

These larger magnets are available encased in plastic and color coded so the two polarities are easily determined. The large neodymium magnets or stronger ferrite magnets are indicated in prescriptions for treating most acute and chronic conditions.

Biomagnetic therapy also consists of systematically laying strong magnetic bars over affected areas for a duration of approximately 30 minutes to an hour, two or three times daily. For many conditions the application of several acu-magnets will be more convenient and often as effective, especially for less serious conditions.

Magnetic Mattresses, Mattress Pads and Pillows

Magnetic mattresses, mattress pads and pillows are designed to provide a sound and restful sleep. The result is that we awaken with more energy, alertness and fewer aches and pains. For those who are bedridden, they powerfully help to prevent bedsores. In general, it is best to use magnetic mattresses or mattress pads with low gauss, alternate North and South facing magnets. Because their intended use is long term, only low gauss magnets (under 1000), should be used.

These products are currently being manufactured by companies throughout Japan and other Asian countries such as China, as well as North America. I have seen them available as top quality, thick full sized mattresses and less expensive mattress pads that can be laid over the top of a preexisting mattress. These can have a beneficial effect for most people but especially for those whose conditions are more systemic, such as individuals suffering from chronic pains such as multiple sclerosis, fibromyalgia, arthritis and rheumatic conditions.

Magnetic pillows and pillow inserts can be used for those who have trouble with insomnia, chronic neck and shoulder aches, those who snore excessively or suffer from sleep apnea (stopped breathing while sleeping). Based on their effects, it is believed that low gauss magnetic pillows and magnetic pillow inserts help to promote the natural secretion of melatonin from the pineal gland. This hormone is important to regulate sleep cycles, counteract jetlag and to serve as an anti-oxidant for the prevention and treatment of various chronic diseases and other conditions associated with aging.

Because the Japanese have had a long history of appreciation for natural health products it is estimated that one out of eight Japanese use a magnetic mattress sleep system. This is further reflected in the lead the Japanese have taken in researching magnets and other natural magnetic products.

A few individuals may experience temporary discomfort when first sleeping on a magnetic sleep system. This is because with greater circulation, more toxins are being flushed out at an increased rate. For these, it may take gradual periodic use over several days or weeks. The time spent acclimatizing to it is worth the investment and provides a significant passive contribution to long term health and wellness. In the resources section at the end of the book there is a list of distributors and suppliers of these and other magnet products.

Magnetized Water and Herb Teas

The proclaimed healing powers of various naturally occurring baths at places such as Lourdes in France, Sedona in Arizona and Jesus Chahin's well in Tlacote, Mexico, occur in areas where there is reportedly higher naturally occurring magnetic energy. One way to naturally magnetize water is to run it through 30 feet of sand where it will emerge negatively poled because of the effect of minute quartz sand crystals. This water emerges saturated with oxygen that is able to kill germs, build bodily strength and support the immune system. Water so treated will show a change of temperature, surface tension, viscosity and electrical conductivity. Just as chemicals change weight after being subjected to magnetic fields, so does water. More hydroxyl (OH-) ions are generated to form calcium bicarbonate and other alkaline particles. Normal water has a pH level of around 7, while magnetized water can reach 9.2 pH after exposure to a 7000 gauss strength magnet. This has been shown to be enough to destroy cancer cells.[7](Barefoot and Reich).

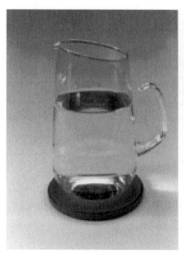 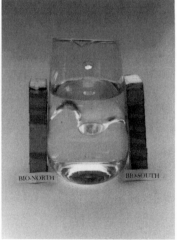

Cancer is practically unknown to the Hopi Indians of Arizona and the Hunza of Pakistan, so long as they drink from their local water supply, which is rich in rubidium and potassium in the case of the Hopi water and rich in caesium and potassium for the Hunza people. The salts of these alkalinizing minerals have the effect of counteracting toxic acidity by raising body pH. Cancer cells are destroyed with an enriched oxygenated environment.

By standing a container of water on either the South or North pole of a magnet for a period of approximately 24 hours, one can imbue it with specific Yin, sedating and dispersing properties or Yang, tonifying and coalescing properties. This water can then be taken internally throughout the day. Water can also be potentized by tying or taping South and North pole magnets to opposite sides of a rectangular bottle or jug.

Herbal teas intended for tonification can be augmented by setting the cup of tea on a South Magnetized surface for an hour or so before drinking. If the tea consists of dispersing, anti-inflammatory or sedative herbs, then the North pole of the magnet should be used. Special magnetic cups and containers for making magnetized water are available from various magnetic product suppliers and Japanese sources.

Magnetic Insoles

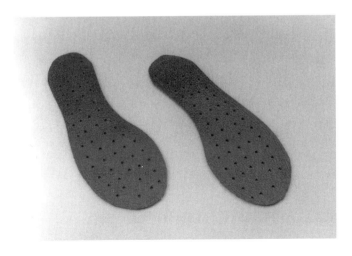

The feet and legs are sometimes called the 'second heart' because return circulation from this area of the body is vital to health. Besides being highly effective for all foot problems (such as diabetic and other neuropathies) the regular use of magnetic insoles increase energy and vitality throughout the day. Like the magnetic bed, wearing these insoles constitutes an effective passive long term investment in one's health.

Magnetic Balls

These are remarkable because while they have a very low gauss strength, when the balls are rapidly revolved or manipulated they shoot their electrons out for some distance into the body. They are available from various distributors and are very useful when vigorously rolled over affected bodily areas to relieve injury and pains. The balls, removed from their holder, rolled between the palms and fingers for 10 minutes or so each day, are very effective to treat stiffness and arthritic pains in the hands and fingers. They are especially useful as a warm-up for pianists and musicians.

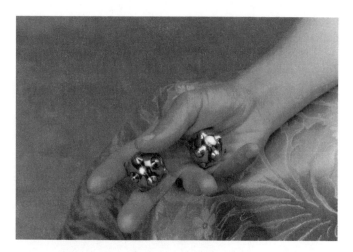

U-shaped or Horseshoe magnets

These are available from industrial magnet manufacturers and may also be found in hardware stores. The two ends are bent into a U shape with one end being South and the other North. They are useful for conditions where the application of a strong bipolar magnetic field is indicated. They can also be used by making slow passes down the spine or another area to improve circulation and relieve pain. Because both ends of the magnet create a magnetic field, these can eventually lose their strength over time. They should be stored with a 'keeper', which is a piece of metal that connects both ends of the magnet.

Electromagnets

These are used by practitioners and hospitals for chronic disease including bone and scar tissue healing, sciatica, arthritis, and sports injuries. Sports therapists were among the first to introduce the use of medical magnets. The combined use of electromagnetic machines with permanent magnets has been found to reduce by half the time required for healing injuries, sprains, tendon and muscle injuries. These machines are especially effective for treating large areas of pain.

Magnetic Jewelry

Necklaces can be used for diseases of the chest, throat, neck, shoulders, sore throat, asthma, irregular heart beat and angina. Bracelets and rings are worn for controlling blood pressure as well as hand and arm pain. They are available in many designs ranging from 700 to 1300 gauss.

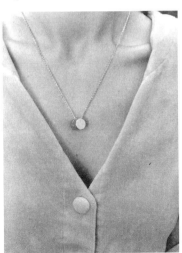 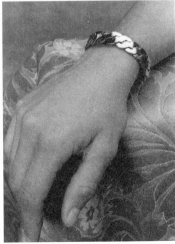

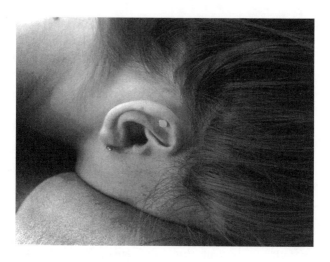

Magnetite or Lodestone

These are naturally occurring magnets associated with a type of iron ore. Generally the Gauss rating is low, from 300 to no more than 700 Gauss. Since ancient times, jewelry in the form of necklaces, bracelets and rings were worn for various therapeutic reasons. The Egyptians believed the magnet had a divine power and wore them to relieve headache, gout, dropsy and to maintain vitality and health. Cleopatra (69-30 BC) supposedly wore a polished lodestone magnet on her forehead to maintain her beauty.

Magnetic Foil

Magnetic foil consists of a low gauss metallic foil that can be cut to various sizes and applied topically over wider areas than acuband magnets. It has been pioneered by a Swedish therapist, Holger Hanneman, for the treatment of 'soft tissue' rheumatism. It seems that this is another variation of the flex magnets previously described.

BIOMAGNETIC TREATMENT OF THE WHOLE BODY

Biomagnetics can be used to treat the body systemically as opposed to their use over specific acupuncture points or what are known as pain or "trigger" points.

There is a difference in the energy between the upper from the lower, the right from the left sides of the body. The area from the chest upwards tends to reflect the more positive, outgoing energy. With imbalance, this can manifest to extreme with symptoms ranging from skin eruptions, mental excitation, eye, ear, nose, throat and lung problems and hypertension. For this reason the North magnet is more frequently indicated in this area to disperse the excess. The lower area of the body, below the umbilicus, is often over-extended upward and needs South or coalescing, grounding energy. The right side of the body is the more positive side and usually gets the North magnet while the left side which is more negative, receives the South magnet. Thus the following configurations have been adopted for systemic treatment:

Diseases above the navel: Place the right hand on the North magnet and the left hand on Bio- South for 15 to 30 minutes.

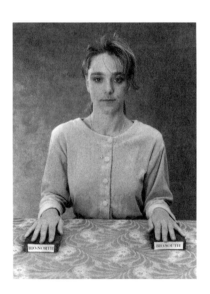

Diseases below the navel: Place the right foot on the North pole and the left foot on the South.

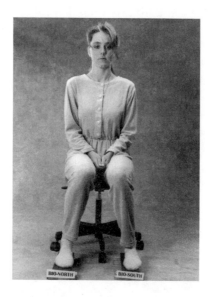

Diseases on the right side of the body: Right hand on the North pole and right foot on the South pole.

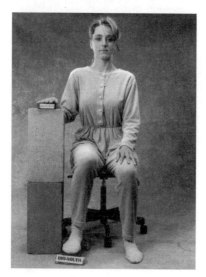

Diseases on the left side of the body: Left hand on the North pole and left foot on the South.

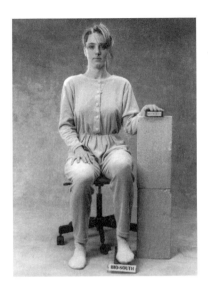

Diseases of the digestive system: Right hand on the North pole and left foot on the South.

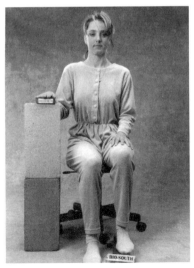

Dietary Treatment

Just as magnets express South or positive energies and North or negative energies, so also do the various foods. This is not the place to enter an exhaustive treatment of food therapy, but one who uses biomagnetic therapy will be able to achieve the most optimal results without negating the effects with inappropriate diet.

Positive Polarity Foods: Animal products, including meat, fish, eggs and dairy, concentrated sugar and spices have warming and stimulating properties and should be left out of the diet entirely or limited when treating diseases associated with excess, inflammation and stagnation.

Negative Polarity Foods: Vegetable products and fruits should be used for excess type diseases, inflammations and stagnations. They should, however, be cooked when there is digestive coldness or weakness.

Balanced Polarity Foods: These include whole grains, beans, cooked vegetables. For treating acute conditions one should select mostly from foods that represent the balanced polarity and limit foods from the positive polarity category.

Four Day Apple Juice Cleansing Fast

Ingredients needed for the fast:

1. At least one half gallon of organic (preferably freshly juiced) apple juice per day.

2. Capsules of cayenne pepper

3. Pure virgin olive oil

4. Triphala

5. Agar Agar flakes (seaweed to maintain electrolyte levels and aid elimination)

Procedure: For three days have only one half glass of apple juice every two hours; one tablespoon of olive oil three times each day; two 00 sized capsules of Cayenne pepper three or more times a day (have Cayenne more often if you are feeling tired); two tablets of Triphala three times daily.

On the fourth day break the fast with warm vegetable broth and continue through the day with finely chopped salads, steamed vegetables seasoned with sea salt, olive oil, lemon juice or unrefined apple cider vinegar.

For the next three days continue with congee brown rice cream or rice porridge. First pan toast the rice to make it more metabolically warming. Cook the rice a long time using one cup of rice to 4 to 7 cups of water. Garnish with toasted and roughly grated sesame seeds (high in protein and calcium). Warm vegetable soups with noodles or rice are appropriate. Use beans, peas, tofu, seitan (wheat gluten) or tempeh for protein complement once or twice a day. Baked fruit and/or apple sauce can be used for dessert. Continue with the Triphala tablets and cayenne capsules.

This is a general detoxifying diet useful for many diseases. For those who are overweight, one can lose 10 to 15 lbs. in a week on this diet.

For those who may find the above diet too cleansing and eliminating or otherwise cannot afford to lose weight, the following may be more appropriate:

The Ten Day Kicharee Diet

Kicharee is an ancient Indian recipe that has been regarded for centuries as being the most healing and balanced food. Tradition in India states that if *Kicharee* is eaten as the sole food for three weeks, all diseases will be cured. It makes a wonderful alternate and complement to the Japanese 10 day brown rice diet, which also utilizes a combination of whole grains and beans as the sole primary food. Both these diets have the effect of balancing blood chemistry, normalizing all physiological processes and centering and calming the mind. As such it is the most balanced and ideal fasting diet to insure the benefits of biomagnetic and herbal therapy.

Kicharee is a combination of equal parts mung beans and brown or basmati rice, cooked with a pinch of sea salt, ghee, coriander, cumin and turmeric powders. During the cold season, dry ginger can be added to maintain metabolism and heat.

To prepare *kicharee*, begin by precooking presoaked mung beans until soft and palatable. Next cook rice and sauté powdered coriander seeds, cumin seeds and turmeric root in a skillet with approximately one tablespoon of ghee (clarified butter) until the spices are lightly toasted. Stir the combined rice and mung beans into the skillet with the ghee and spices. *Kicharee* can be thicker and more solid or thinner by adding water. Variations can be made by adding cooked vegetables to make it more of a stew.

Kicharee is a complete protein and whole food that one can live on for months as a sole diet. Unlike other protein sources, mung beans neutralize acids and actually detoxify the blood. This food is ideal to use to lower and regulate high blood pressure. *Kicharee* is a good fast to either do alone or to follow the initial 3 day apple juice fast described above.

Homeopathic Treatment
Homeopathy was evolved by Dr. Samuel Hahnemann out of his dissatisfaction with the allopathic system of medicine practiced during his time. While it is doubtful that he would be any more satisfied with the way it is practiced today, we have come to a crossroad where all medical systems can work together to provide the best medical options for all people.

Homeopathy is based on the laws of potentization and similars. As we shall see, both of these have a close affinity with the principles of biomagnetism. Potentization is based on subjecting a diluted drug substance to processes known as 'shock succussion' (in alcohol) or 'trituration' (in milk-sugar powder) with the medicine increasing in potency and effectiveness with higher and higher dilutions. In potencies above the 30th, there is no indication of any drug substance remaining, yet the medicine seems to continue to become stronger even to the millionth potency.

The law of similars describes how a homeopathic drug is chosen based on its ability, in gross crude form, to produce the symptoms similar to that of a specific disease. Thus if the symptoms of the drug somehow mimics certain disease symptoms, it would fit the similamum and would be used homeopathically in high dilutions to treat the disease. This is similar to the principle of immunization, except that immunization as it is practiced uses quantifiable disease material, hopefully neutralized and sterilized, and then injected directly into the blood.

Homeopathy uses only the biomagnetic energy of a substance. This would allow for the use of a variety of familiar medicinal herbs, including poisonous plants like aconite, poisonous insect and snake venom as well as common articles such as the onion or table salt for homeopathic preparations.

According to contemporary investigation, the processes of succussion or trituration disturb the atomic state of a drug substance by jolting an electron (negative charge) into a higher orbit. This disturbance of the electron-proton balance of the atom causes it to release its characteristic electro-magnetic wave, which accounts for its therapeutic effects.

Like all systems of healing, that which can cure can also kill. Just as we should be careful of inappropriately subjecting the body to high strength magnets over a prolonged period, we should also refrain from the use of high potency homeopathic preparations without considerable study. All the indications given in the following section, therefore, should be for preparations that are no higher than the 30th potency.

The basis of homeopathy has thus far confounded gross scientific investigative methods, yet it continues to be practiced with great effectiveness and growing appreciation throughout the world.

Herbal Medicine

Herbal medicine is the oldest system of medicine on the planet. Unlike homeopathy, herbs provide a substantial connection between food and medicine because they possess many of the same micro-nutrients as food such as vitamins, minerals and special substances currently recognized as 'phyto-nutrients'.

In the following sections, out of convenience, I have given the simplest and most effective herbal remedies for specific conditions. I have also indicated proprietary Planetary formulas which evolved out of years of personal clinical practice. One can select either or use both in combination, which may have an even better effect.

METHODS OF TAKING HERBS
How to Make An Herb Tea

Use good quality fresh or freshly dried herbs. Prepare in non-metallic containers such as glass, earthenware or enamel pots. Stainless steel is acceptable when these others are not available.

The dose is important. For medicinal tea, the dose is at least *one ounce of the combined herbs to a pint of water (two cups)*. If fresh herbs are used, use one and one half to two ounces of herbs to the same amount of water. An ounce of most dried herbs is usually around a handful of material, more or less depending upon density and weight. Whenever possible, use distilled or spring water.

There are basically two methods for preparing herb teas. One is the decoction method that is suitable for heavier roots, barks and non-volatile (non-odorous) plants. Here the water is brought to a rolling boil and the herbs are added; the fire is turned down to a simmer which is to continue for anywhere from 20 to 45 minutes on a low flame.

The second infusion method is for volatile lighter leaves and flowers. Here the water is brought to a rolling boil and poured over the herbs. The pot is immediately covered and taken off the flame entirely and allowed to infuse for 10 to 20 minutes or until cool enough to drink.

The average adult dose is one cup two or three times a day. Children (under 12) are given half or less according to age and tolerance.

Herbal Powders and Pills
Here the herb is powdered and pressed into gelatin capsules or pills. This method is particularly convenient for long term compliance since the bitter taste of many medicinal herbs can be a hindrance to regular usage. A smaller dose is usually required for chronic treatment so that smaller amounts of herbal powders are indicated. On the average, one should take an adult dose of anywhere from four to six grams of powdered herb in a day. Depending on the size of the capsule or pill, this averages out to around two capsules or pills threes times a day, ideally with warm water. Children under 12 years should be given less according to age.

This is usually the minimum dose, and if it is well tolerated in most cases it can be at least doubled or even tripled as a specific complaint is targeted for treatment. If the pill or powder is being used for an acute condition such as a fever, cold or influenza, more should be taken approximately every two hours, with the dose being tapered off as symptoms begin to subside.

Herbal powders are more easily given to children since they can be mixed with honey or maple syrup.

Tinctures

Tinctures depend upon a combination of alcohol and water to extract the active constituents of an herb. Besides being an extractive agent and easy to absorb, the alcohol acts as a long time preservative so that most tinctures are good for at least three years. They are also very convenient to use which makes them commercially popular. For some with an alcohol intolerance or who may be concerned about the negative influence of even a small amount of alcohol in relation to liver toxicity, this may not be a satisfactory way to take herbs. The choice is to use teas, capsules or pills or place the requisite amount of tincture in a cup of boiling water for a few minutes, which will help to evaporate a large portion of the alcoholic content.

It is quite easy to make one's own herbal tincture using vodka, gin or some other spirits. Simply macerate at least four ounces of the powdered or finely cut herb in the alcoholic menstruum for at least two weeks or more (it can be for several months). Again double the amount would be better for tincturing fresh herbs to account for their high water content. Always use a wide necked container to ease removing the contents later.

After the required period of time, press-strain the herbs through a fine cloth and store the liquor for use. The average adult dose for most medicinal tinctures is anywhere from a half to one teaspoon (30 to 60 drops) two or three times a day. Again it is taken more frequently for acute ailments.

Syrups

Syrups are made with a base of sugar syrup, honey or perhaps maple syrup. There are various ways to make them but for the purposes of this book the simplest is to blend the mashed herb (such as onion or garlic), the herbal tincture, or powder with honey. A good basic cough syrup can be made with honey, lemon and onions or garlic.

Liniments and Oils

These are intended for external use to treat bruises, injuries or soft tissue pains. Liniments can be made with alcohol or vinegar. Jethro Kloss' All-Purpose Liniment is a good one to begin with. Combine one ounce each of Golden seal, Myrrh gum and a half ounce of Cayenne pepper in a quart of vinegar. Cover tightly, shake the mixture once each day for at least 7 days, then strain and bottle for use.

Oils are made by impregnating a basic oil such as olive oil or sesame oil with an herb. There are various methods. One can add an amount of herbal tincture to the oil and heat until all the alcohol and water is evaporated away. This is not so effective if one is attempting to capture active volatile constituents such as essential oils. Chickweed oil, which is a good lotion for skin ailments, is made by placing an ounce of dried chickweed in olive oil. Heat gently for awhile until the oil takes on a somewhat 'greener' appearance. Allow to cool then strain and bottle for use. Garlic oil is quickly made by blending fresh garlic cloves in olive oil. This can be strained or used with the mash.

Herbal oils can be further potentized by exposing them to the effects of bio-north magnetic field (for trauma and inflammation) or bio-south magnetic field (for strengthening, warming and tonification) for at least 24 hours prior to use. (See magnetized water.)

TREATMENT PROTOCOLS
FOR SPECIFIC CONDITIONS

Abscess
Apply a North seeking or low gauss bipolar magnet to the affected site.

Herbal: A combination of tincture of Echinacea and Golden Seal internally and externally applied.

Planetary Formula: River of Life, Echinacea, Cat's Claw Complex

Homeopathic: Silicea, Hepar Sulph.

Acidity
Apply North pole or bipolar magnets to the abdomen. Drink North 'magnetized' water.

Herbal: Use Marshmallow root and Chickweed tea or strong Chamomile tea.

Homeopathic: Natrum Phos

Acne (see Skin)

Allergies (upper respiratory and sinus congestion)
Apply North acuband magnets to both sides of the nostrils. Apply North magnets to the chest and upper back.

Herbal: Ephedra, Eyebright

Planetary formula: Breeze Free

Homeopathic: Silicea, Kali Bichromicum

Alopecia
Use North seeking or bipolar magnets on the scalp. Make Castor and Cayenne pepper oil by heating a cup of castor oil with one teaspoon of Cayenne pepper extract and four teaspoons of Prickly Ash extract until the alcohol is evaporated. Let this cool for at least 24 hours while being exposed to the North seeking side of a magnet. The oil is ready for use and should be vigorously rubbed on the scalp an hour before showering each day, or for faster results two or three times daily. After applying the oil, purchase a

seven star dermal hammer from an acupuncture supply distributor and lightly tap various areas of the scalp with the dermal hammer.

Herbal: Internally use blood and circulatory tonics such as Angelica root and Juniper berries.

Planetary Formula: Women's Treasure (for men also) and Yin Energetics

Homeopathic: Acidum Fluoricum, Acidum Phosphoricum, Selenium.

Anemia

First determine and treat the underlying cause which may be hemorrhage or imbalanced nutrition. Use a bipolar magnetic mattress and drink water exposed to both the North and South poles.

Herbal: Use Cayenne pepper internally to stop hemorrhage. For counteracting anemia make a combination tea of 9 grams astragalus root, 3 grams of Dang gui (Angelica sinensis) and 6 grams Yellow Dock root. Take three times daily. If possible eat organ meats such as organic liver.

Planetary Formula: Women's Treasure (also for men) and/or Eight Precious Herbs

Homeopathic: Calcarea Phosphate, Ferum Phosphate and Natrum Mur.

Anorexia

South or bipolar magnet over the umbilicus and/or stomach area. South magnet over the spine opposite the navel (acupoint Governor 4). Drink bipolar magnetized water.

Herbal: Bitters containing Gentian, Goldenseal, Calamus, Juniper and Ginger. Ginger and Ginseng tea.

Planetary Formula: Planetary Bitters formula

Homeopathic: Nux Vomica, China

Angina

North magnet over the heart. South pole magnet or bracelet to the right wrist. Drink South magnetized water.

Herbal: Cayenne pepper, Hawthorn berries, Chinese Red Sage root (Salvia miltiorrhiza)

Planetary Formula: Life Pulse

Homeopathic: Ferrum Phos

Apoplexy (stroke)

Apply a North or bipolar magnet to the center of the forehead. North magnets along the spine to disperse the stagnation. South pole magnet or bracelet to the right wrist. Depending on the hemisphere of the head that is affected, apply North pole or bipolar magnets to the affected hemisphere of the head.

Appendicitis

Do not try to treat acute appendicitis as there is a grave risk of it bursting; that could cause massive abdominal inflammation and death. For chronic appendicitis, apply a North or bipolar magnet over the affected area of the abdomen.

Arthritis and Rheumatic Complaints

Apply bipolar or North magnet to the affected area(s). Sleeping on a magnetic mattress can be very helpful. Rolling magnetic balls in the hand or other parts of the body regularly is very effective for arthritic conditions, especially in the hands and fingers.

The principle is that when there is inflammation use the North seeking magnet; for degeneration of the bones and tissues, perhaps the South seeking magnet will be more effective, or a combination of both. Bipolar magnets make unnecessary the need to decide when to use either the North or South.

In any case, as with any pains, magnetic therapy is one of the most effective methods of achieving relatively fast relief with approximately 90% effectiveness.

Herbal: Make a tea combining Sarsaparilla, Burdock root, Sassafras, Poke root, Prickly ash, Black Cohosh and Ginger. Take three cups daily.

Planetary Formula: Flexibility tonic

Homeopathic: Rhus Tox, Bryonia, Causticum, Caulophyllum, Ledum Pal., Sulfur

Arteriosclerosis
Drink water exposed to both North and South polarities.

Herbal: Cayenne pepper or Garlic

Planetary Formula: Guggul

Homeopathic: Arsenic iod., Baryta Carb., Calcarea Fluor., Crataegus

Ascites or Edema
Drink water exposed to both magnetic poles.

Asthma (bronchial)
Apply a large bipolar flex magnet to the back or chest. Drink water that has been exposed to both poles.

Herbal: Ma Huang (Ephedra), Mullein, Comfrey leaf, Wild Cherry Bark, a half part Lobelia leaf and Ginger.

Planetary Formula: Breeze Free

Homeopathic: Arsenicum Album, Ipecac, Spongia, Thuja, Senega

Atrophy (Muscular)
Apply South magnets to the affected muscles.

Back Pain (Lower) (also sciatica and lumbago)
Apply North or bipolar magnets to the affected area.

Herbal: Loranthes (Chinese herb called "Sang Ji Sheng"), simmer 15 grams in 3 cups of boiling water down to two. Have two cups daily.

Planetary Formula: Back-Ease

Homeopathic: Rhus Tox or Bryonia

Bell's Palsy

Apply the South pole magnet to the affected muscle of the face and the seventh cranial nerve behind the ear on the same side.

North pole can be applied to the lower jaw of the affected side and the South pole to the affected cheek or facial muscles.

Homeopathic: Aconite Napellus upon immediate onset of symptoms followed by Caustic, Ammonium Phosphoric or Rhus Tox.

Biliousness

Apply the North pole to the affected abdominal region. Drink North magnetized water.

Herbal: Chamomile tea

Planetary: Digestive Comfort

Homeopathic: Nux Vomica, Chelidonium, Natrum Sulph, Bryonia

Blood Pressure, Reducing or Raising

To reduce blood pressure, wear a bipolar magnetized bracelet on the right wrist. To raise it, wear it on the left wrist.

Another method is to place a small North magnet under the right ear along the carotid artery.

For either type, drink water exposed to both magnetic poles.

Herbal: Use Hawthorn berries and leaf extract with Garlic.

Planetary Formula: Life Pulse

Bronchitis and Sore Throat

Apply North pole magnets to the base of the throat and over both sides of the lungs. North Acuband magnets can be placed an inch and a half alongside the spine between the 2nd and 3rd thoracic vertebrae of the back.

North magnets can also be applied to the Hegu point (Colon 4) on the dorsal surface of the hand between the thumb and 2nd finger.

Herbal: A tea of equal parts Mullein, Yerba Santa, Echinacea and Licorice can be taken.

Planetary Formula: Cat's Claw Complex

Homeopathic: Arsenicum Album, Bryonia, Ipecac, Antimonium Tart., Senega

Burns

To treat local or limited burn areas, apply the North directly over the burn area for 30 to 45 minutes 2 or 3 times a day. North magnetized water can be used over the area as well. When it begins to scab over, use the South to promote faster healing and repair with little or no scarring.

Herbal: Apply Aloe Vera Gel or a salve of Calendula and/or Comfrey.

Homeopathic: Causticum, Urtica Urens

Cancer

Regular application of high gauss North seeking pole magnets has been effective in checking the growth and occasionally shrinking tumors. Here Dr. Wollin's experience with high gauss neodymium magnets is specifically indicated. It is recommended to apply the North magnet over the area for a half hour at a time, three times daily. At the same time North magnetized water should be drunk. Skin cancers respond well to the topical application of strong North magnets.

Herbs: Red Clover, Chaparral, Poke root and Burdock root tea should be taken three times daily; for skin cancers paint on Bloodroot tincture.

Planetary Formulas: Complete Pau d' Arco and Cat's Claw Complex

Cholesterol, High

Drink water exposed to the North or bipolar poles.

Chronic fatigue, Fibromyalgia

Use a magnetic bed, magnetic insoles and individual bipolar magnets on the sites of discomfort. For insomnia, apply a North magnet, around 1000 gauss, between the eyebrows for 10 to 15 minutes before retiring.

Constipation
Apply North or bipolar magnet to the lower abdominal region. Drink bipolar water.

Herbal: Rhubarb, cascara, buckthorne, senna leaves, psyllium husk.

Planetary: Triphala

Homeopathic: Nux Vomica, Alumen, Bryonia, Alumina

Cystitis
Apply North or bipolar magnet over the pubic region. Drink North magnetized water.

Herbal: Tea or powder of cherry stems; another choice is a tea of Uva Ursi, Buchu, Parsley leaf and Marshmallow root.

Planetary Formula: Diurite with a tincture of Golden seal and Echinacea.

Diabetes:
Use magnetic insoles regularly along with the magnetic mattress pad. According to experiments by Dr. Roy Davis, the application of the South magnet to the pancreas for approximately 30 minutes morning and evening "appeared to have either raised the amount of insulin produced by the pancreas or strengthened it to a point where less positive blood sugars were noted when samples were taken and tested for sugars in the urine". Drink bipolar magnetized water.

Herbal: One teaspoon of turmeric powder in capsules three times daily

Planetary formula: Energetics Yin

Homeopathic: Arsenicum Album, Bromide, Acid Phosphoricum.

Diarrhea
Apply bipolar or North magnet to the lower left abdominal region.

Herbal: Cranesbill root, Agrimony, Oak bark and Blackberry root bark

Planetary formula: Digestive Comfort

Dysentery

Same treatment as for diarrhea.

Herbal: Use similar herbs as above but add golden seal and garlic along with a rice fast.

Planetary formula: Digestive Comfort and Triphala

Homeopathic: Mercurius, Aloe, Nux Vomica

Ears

1. Inflammation

Use North magnets on or around the ear.

Herbal: Garlic and Olive oil drops in the ears or Rue oil is effective. Internally take Echinacea and Golden seal extract.

Homeopathic: Aconite, Hepar Sulph., Pulsatilla

2. **Deafness**

Understand the cause. If the ears are plugged with wax, have it removed by a specialist or try using ear candles. If deafness is caused by inflammation, use the North Magnet. If it is caused by degeneration, use alternating North and South magnets.

3. **Ringing** (as in Meniere's)

Apply a North magnet bar over each ear, 20 to 30 minutes 2 or 3 times daily.

Herbal: Ginger compress

Eyes

Conjunctivitis, Cataract, Glaucoma and other disorders: Apply North or bipolar magnets over the closed eyelids for at least a half hour three times daily.

Fever

Apply North pole to the forehead and lower abdomen. Drink North magnetized water.

Herbal: Tea of Yarrow, Feverfew, Lemon Balm and Peppermint
Homeopathic: Aconite, Belladonna

Fracture (non-healing)

1. Apply bipolar magnets over the affected area

2. Apply alternate North and South magnets along the affected area.

3. Apply a strong North Magnet to one end of the injury and South to the other end.

Herbal: Comfrey root tea

Homeopathic: Calcarea Phosphate, Symphytum

Flatulence

Apply South pole magnet to the umbilicus and lower abdomen. Drink bipolar magnetized water.

Herbal: Anise seeds, Fennel seeds

Planetary Formula: Hingashtak

Homeopathic: Cinchona, Lycopodium, Magnesium Phosphoricum.

Gallstones

Apply a North or bipolar magnet to the affected area. Drink bipolar magnetized water.

Herbal: Turmeric root, one teaspoon three times daily.

Planetary Formula: Stone Free

Case: Woman, age 65, diagnosed with acute abdominal pains. She was recommended by her doctor to surgery to remove her gallstones. Besides taking Stone Free formula, she underwent the four day cleansing fast with apple juice, olive oil, cayenne pepper and triphala. After this she went on a balanced diet of whole grains, beans, occasional fish and other range fed animal products, vegetables and fruit, while abstaining strictly from sugar, coffee, refined foods with additives, and dairy products. Acuband North magnets (9000 gauss) were applied to the most sensitive areas on her abdomen and left on for two weeks. The first week her pains were somewhat aggravated. The second week she returned completely pain free, feeling better than she ever had before.

Gynecology:
1. Amenorrhea (Suppressed menses)

Apply South pole or bipolar magnets to the pubic region.

Herbal: Tea of Angelica root, Black and Blue Cohosh, Squaw Vine and Wild Ginger.

Planetary Formula: Women's Treasure

(All menstrual irregularities should be treated herbally for at least three months to accommodate the alternation between the right and left ovary).

Homeopathic: Pulsatilla, Natrum Muriaticum

2. Dysmenorrhea (Painful Menstruation)
Apply North or bipolar magnet to the lower abdomen.

Herbal: Warm application of Castor oil to the abdomen, with a flannel cloth lightly saturated with fresh ginger tea placed over the area, and a heating pad. Drink a tea of Chamomile and Ginger.

Planetary Formulas: Women's Treasure or Women's Comfort with Emotional Balance and Hepato Pure

3. Menorrhagia (Excessive Menstruation)
Usually, this is more of an inflamed condition and one should apply the North or bipolar magnets to the pubic region or perineum.

Herbal: Tea of two parts Vitex berries and one part each of Raspberry leaf, Squaw vine, Bethroot, False Unicorn and Cramp Bark.

Planetary Formula: Emotional Balance

Homeopathic: Ipecac, Trillium, Sepia

4. Infertility:
South or bipolar magnet to the pubic region.

Herbal: False Unicorn root, Black Haw or Cramp Bark and Raspberry leaf .

Planetary Formula: Women's Treasure

5. Leukorrhea
Apply North pole magnet to the perineum or pubic region. Bipolar magnetized water should be taken regularly.

Herbal: Douche with garlic tea to which is added three tablespoons of acidophilus yogurt.

Planetary Formula: Hepato Pure, Women's Treasure

Homeopathic: Sepia, Pulsatilla, Alumina, Kreosote

Hemorrhoids
Sit on a North pole magnet. A seat cushion with magnets is very effective for this purpose.

Herbal: A suppository made of Collinsonia root or a combination of the powders of Bayberry bark, Yarrow, Prickly Ash, Oak Bark and Slippery Elm can be mixed with cocoa butter and inserted each evening.

Planetary: Triphala

Headache
Apply bipolar magnets to the temples.

Herbal: Feverfew, Rosemary, White Willow bark

Planetary: Head-Aid

Heart problems (see Angina)

Impotence
Apply a South pole magnet to the pubic region.

Herbal: Ginseng, Epimedium, Damiana, Yohimbe

Planetary: Male Potential, Wu Zi Wan, Energetics Yang

Inflammations (see Septic Conditions)

Influenza (same treatment as for Rhinitis)

Insomnia
Apply a North magnet to the center of the forehead for ten minutes before retiring. Sleep on a magnetic mattress. Place a North pole magnet face up under the pillow each night.

Herbal: Valerian, Passion Flower, Skullcap

Planetary Formulas: Easy Sleep or Stress Free

Homeopathic: Coffea, Kali Phos.

Kidney Stones

Place a bipolar magnet and/or a combination of North and South pole acuband magnets (at least 3000 gauss) directly over the right or left lumbar area of the lower back, depending on which area is affected. A U shaped magnet can be applied over affected area for approximately an hour once or twice a day.

Herbal: A combination tea of equal parts Hydrangea root, Uva Ursi, Parsley root, Gravel root with a half part each of Marshmallow root and Ginger should be taken three times daily.

Planetary Formula: Stone Free and Diurite

Homeopathic: Berberis vulgaris, Sarsaparilla, Lycopodium

Laryngitis

Apply a North pole magnet to the larynx. This can also be used to improve the singing voice.

Liver Diseases (Cirrhosis, Hepatitis and Jaundice)

Apply North or bipolar magnets over the right hypochondriac region. Drink South magnetized water.

Herbal: Dandelion root, Milk Thistle seed, Wild Yam, Barberry root and Fennel seed tea or a tea of artichoke leaves.

Planetary Formula: Hepato Pure

Homeopathic: Chelidonium, Mercurius

Lumbago

Apply bipolar or North magnets to the 'trigger' points on the back. Roll magnetic balls once or twice a day over the affected area.

Herbal: Comfrey root tea

Planetary formula: Energetics Yang and Energetics Yin

Homeopathic: Rhus Tox., Bryonia, Nux Vomica, Kali Carbonicum

Lung Problems (see Asthma)

This includes a wide range of problems including asthma, pleurisy, emphysema. In general, to remove congestion apply North magnets to the back and/or chest. A Bipolar magnet offers very good results for most people.

Multiple Sclerosis

Sleeping on a magnetized mattress is specifically indicated. The head especially should be exposed to the North pole. Two magnets between 1000 and 2000 gauss should be kept under the pillow. Use a U shaped magnet and pass it slowly down the spine once or twice daily. The North removes the spasms while the South increases strength and regeneration. Drink bipolar water.

Muscle Strain and Cramps

Apply North magnets to the affected areas to relieve tension. Roll magnetic balls over the affected area as frequently as you can.

Nausea

Drink bipolar magnetized water.

Herbal: Ginger

Homeopathic: Ipecac, Nux Vomica, Tabacum, Petroleum and Cocculus for car and sea sickness.

Neuralgia

Similar to arthritic and rheumatic complaints. Apply North magnet to the affected nerves. Drink North magnetized water. Roll magnetic balls over the area frequently.

Herbal: Black Cohosh, White Willow bark, Angelica root tea.

Planetary Formula: Narayana Oil applied externally, Flexibility Tonic

Neurasthenia (Nervous Debility)

The North magnet is both anti-inflammatory and soothing. Apply the North to the head and the South on the lower back or below the umbilicus to 'ground' the energy below.

Herbal: Skullcap, Lady's Slipper

Planetary formula: Stress Free

Homeopathic: Kali Phos., Nux Vomica, Natrum Mur., Argentum

Neuropathies

Similar to Arthritic and Rheumatic problems. If the problem is in the feet, use magnetic insoles.

Osteoporosis

Many astronauts were found to suffer from osteoporosis. This established a better understanding of the role magnetic energy played with calcium and phosphate metabolism. Sleeping on a magnetized mattress and wearing magnetized insoles may be very beneficial to treat and prevent this condition along with appropriate nutritional supplementation. Drinking bipolar magnetized water is also beneficial.

Herbal: Comfrey, Alfalfa and Horsetail

Planetary formulas: Energetics Yin, Energetics Yang and Wu Zi Wan

Parkinson's and Chorea

The North magnet to the cerebral region to help reduce muscular rigidity and tremors. The North magnet can also be passed slowly down the spinal column. Drink magnetized water.

Herbal: Lobelia, Black Cohosh and Skullcap tincture can be taken three times daily.

Planetary Formula: Stress Free

Homeopathic: Aurum Sul., Agaricus, Mercurius

Prostate

To increase prostatic fluid, sit on a South pole for about 30 minutes twice a day.

Herbal: Saw Palmetto, Pygeum, Pumpkin seeds
Planetary formula: Saw Palmetto Complex
Homeopathic: Sabal Serulata, Thuja

Raynaud's Disease (cold extremities)
 Use South magnets at the extremities to increase circulation and remove the vasoconstriction. Drink South magnetized water. Apply the South magnet to the sacrum.

Herbal: Prickly ash, Cayenne, Ginger, Lobelia

Planetary formula: Herbal Uprising, Stress Free

Homeopathic: Arsenicum Album

Rheumatism (see arthritis)

Rhinitis (Common cold and Influenza)
 Use the North magnet over affected areas of the upper respiratory tract. Two North acuband magnets placed on each side of the nostrils will help clear the sinuses. A North magnet placed in the notch at the base of the throat will help control coughing.

Herbal: Yarrow, Lemon Balm, Elder Flowers and Peppermint tea.

Planetary formula: Yin Chiao and Yin Chiao Plus, also Cat's Claw Complex and Echinacea; for coughs use Old Indian Cough Syrup.

Homeopathic: Arsenicum

Ringworm
 Apply North magnets to the affected area.

Herbal: Paint the affected areas with a tincture of Garlic and Walnut husk. Bloodroot tincture is also very useful for this. Frequent cleansing of the area and change of clothes is essential.

Sarcoma
 Use strong neodymium North magnets over the affected area, three times a day, 30 minutes each time.

Herbal: Use Bloodroot tincture topically, Pau d' Arco, Chaparral, Red Clover and Burdock root tea

Planetary formulas: River of Life and Complete Pau d'Arco

Sciatica (see Back Pain or Lumbago)

Septic Conditions and Inflammations

Apply North magnets to the area. Drink North magnetized water.

Herbal: Echinacea, Baptisia and Goldenseal

Planetary formulas: Echinacea and Cat's Claw Complex

Homeopathic: Hepar Sulph., Silicea

Shingles (Herpes Zoster)

Apply the North magnet to the affected area. Drink North magnetized water. Roll magnetic balls lightly and rapidly over the area.

Herbal: Garlic and Olive oil rubbed over the affected area is useful.

Planetary formula: Cat's Claw Complex

Homeopathic: Cantharis, Kalmia latifolia, Mezerum and Ranunculus Bulbosus.

Skin

Skin diseases such as eczema, acne and psoriasis respond very well to the application of North facing or low gauss bipolar magnets. One method is to apply a fine cotton or linen cloth over the affected area and lay a North facing magnet over the site(s) for 30 minutes once or twice a day. Besides their local effect, magnets extend out to benefit the surrounding tissue. For facial acne, apply North seeking magnets to the cheeks and forehead. Acuband magnets can be used if they are convenient. Regular use of magnetic balls rolled over the problem areas is also very effective.

Herbal: Burdock root and seed, Yellow Dock root, Sarsaparilla and Red Clover taken together as a powder or tea three times a day is very effective for clearing the skin. Topical relief can be achieved with Chickweed-Olive oil rubbed over the affected area.

Planetary formula: HerbaDerm and River of Life Complex

Spleen (enlargement as well as enlargement of the liver and lymph glands)

For any enlargement of the Spleen, Liver or Lymph glands one should use the North magnet and drink North magnetized water. It is a good idea to seek proper medical advice to determine the underlying cause.

Herbal and Homeopathic: Ceanothus

Tachycardia and Heart Palpitations

Wear a South bracelet on the right wrist and North magnet over the praecordial region. A magnetic necklace has been effective in cases when all else failed.

Herbal: Hawthorn, Garlic and Cayenne pepper

Planetary formula: Life Pulse

Homeopathic: Abies Nigra, Crataegus

Tennis Elbow

Apply bipolar magnets to the area with an elbow wrap bandage. North magnets are effective over the most painful areas.

Herbal: Liniment made with Golden seal powder, Myrrh, Cayenne pepper and apple cider vinegar applied frequently to the affected area.

Planetary formula: Use Flexibility Tonic as a liniment.

Homeopathic: Rhus Tox., Hypericum and Bryonia

Thyroid (including goiter)

For hyperthyroid, apply a North magnet to the thyroid area to slow down overall activity. Drink North magnetized water.

For hypothyroid, apply a South Magnet to the thyroid area of the neck. Drink South magnetized water.

Both thyroid conditions would benefit from the regular use of a magnetic necklace.

Herbal: Kelp tablets for low thyroid, which is also useful to regulate high thyroid as well, but Bugleweed is specific for treating hyperthyroid.

Planetary Formula: For hypothyroid use Tai Chi formula.

Homeopathic: For hyperthyroid give homeopathic Thyroidinum, Iodum. For hypothyroid give Thyroidinum, Calcarea Carb.

Tinnitus Aurium (Ringing in the ears, see Ears)

Tonsillitis (also called Quinsy)
Apply North magnets to the affected sites of the throat and swollen lymph glands.

Herbal: Echinacea, Golden Seal and Baptisia taken together as an extract is effective.

Trigeminal Neuralgia
Apply bipolar magnets to the affected area or North acuband magnets.

Herbal: Apply Myrrh, Golden Seal, Cayenne in apple cider vinegar frequently to the affected areas.

Planetary formula: Use Flexibility tonic internally and topically as a liniment.

Homeopathic: Right side of the face use Aconitum Napellus, Colocynth, Spigelia or Verbascum.

For the Left side of the face use Cactus Grandiflorus, Coffea, Kalmia, Magnesia Phosphorica, Mezerum.

Ulcer (gastric and duodenal)
Apply North magnets over the site of pain. Drink North magnetized water.

Veins, Varicose
Apply North magnets to affected areas using acuband or other types as convenient.

Herbal: Apply a tincture of Witch Hazel or Bayberry bark and Prickly Ash topically.

Homeopathic: Haemamelis, Calcarea Fluor., Pulsatilla

Vomiting (see Nausea)

Warts

Apply the North pole topically to the area.

Homeopathic: Thuja and Antimonium Tartaricus is very effective. Take alternately two doses of each for 3 days. Repeat consecutively every three weeks three or four times. The warts will disappear.

MISCELLANEOUS USE OF MAGNETS

1. Negating the toxic effects of chemicals, sprays and preservatives from food and water.

Using a strong neodymium magnet, pass it over the food or water 7 times with the North or negative facing downwards.

Follow this by passing the positive South magnet 7 times to energize the food and water and make it easier to digest and absorb.

2. Purifying house water with 2 or 4 magnets.

Fasten one or two (depending on the size of the pipe) negative, North magnets against the water pipe leading into the house. Approximately 2 inches higher, fasten one or two positive South magnets. These can be taped to the water pipes.

According to Dr. Albert Roy Davis, water treated in this way showed little appreciable difference in terms of mineral content, solids, pH or other factors. Testing for the relative amounts of hydrogen and oxygen, it was found that the oxygen level was lower in the treated water as compared with the untreated. While hydrogen amounts were the same, the hydrogen ions were altered to present a much higher degree of activity. This was checked repeatedly with the same findings.

Water treated with either North or South magnetic field tended to reduce the nitrogen in the water, preventing it from going stale. This made it safer for both human consumption and for aquarium fish for a longer period.

3. Potentizing seeds.

Dr. Davis discovered that seeds, exposed to the magnetic force fields of the South pole for anywhere from 6 to 200 hours, showed an improved germination and growth rate, with hardier plants and higher yield of fruit or vegetable products. Exposing seeds to the influence of the North magnetic polarity field resulted in thin, tall plants with poor yields. A simple method is to presoak seeds by placing them in a dish or cup with water on top of a South facing magnet for 24 hours or so before planting.

Fuel Economy

In addition to the above, there are various magnetic devices that can be fixed to the combustion system of automobile engines to economize fuel production. A five star resort in Kawai, Hawaii, installed magnets on the natural gas system of their multimillion dollar units and found that they were able to save $60,000 a year because the gas burned cleaner.

APPENDIX

YOGA AND AYURVEDA AND LAW OF POLARITY

An interesting book called *Magnet Therapy: Theory and Practice* by Dr. Neville S. Bengali (reprinted by Jain in 1986) is very authoritative but seems to confusingly indicate exact opposite effects for the South and North magnetic fields. In this book, Dr. Neville describes the application of magnet therapy through the chakras. The chakras are vortices of energy or nerve plexuses that lie along the spine (while they are depicted along the spine they are actually midway between the medial aspect of the posterior and anterior part of the body). Dr. Neville's use of the magnets on the chakras offers another very effective model for magnetic therapy that deserves to be considered and employed therapeutically.

To begin, we need to outline some of the important aspects of yogic philosophy. The expression of dynamic polarity and magnetism is also described in Ayurvedic medicine and Yogic philosophy as Shiva (positive) and Shakti (negative). Prana is equivalent to the TCM definition of 'Qi' or 'life force'. All concepts imply the unity of energy with breath, but Prana points to a more explicit connection.

It is necessary at this point to briefly diverge to elucidate some basic terms and concepts of Yoga and Ayurveda. The polar expression of the main circulating channels of Prana in the body is described as 'ida' (negative) and 'pingala' (positive). These correspond to the position of the Governor and Conception vessels in acupuncture.

Chakras, as vortices of energy or what are known as 'grand nadis', are similar but more inclusive than acupoints in TCM. Nadis are equivalent to Chinese acupuncture points but Ayurveda maintains that there are 72,000 nadis located throughout the body. There are seven primary chakras located along the spine that correspond to vital TCM acupoints. These will be individually described later at more length.

The dynamic relationship between Ida and Pingala, as with all other fundamental living processes, is based on magnetism; this is described in Western physiology as the sympathetic and para-sympathetic nervous systems. Taoist priests and yogis learned centuries ago that one could influence and control the negative and positive energies of the body through controlling the flow of breath through the right and left nostrils.

An entire system of 'swar' yogic therapy exists based on the breath. There is a natural cycle that occurs frequently through the day where the breath is stronger from either the right or left nostril, corresponding to the alternating of the sympathetic and para-sympathetic nervous systems. When disease first begins, one should use a glass to see which nostril is opened more and place a cotton ball in it. This will prevent the onset of the disease.

To describe further, ida corresponds to the left side of the body and crosses the spinal chord (Sushumna) at various chakras or energy centers and finally at the left nostril to enter the right side of the brain. Pingala governs the right side of the body and transcends various chakras to cross over to the left side of the brain at the nostrils. Kundalini, which is responsible for higher consciousness, cannot ascend the sushumna nadi (channel) from the base (muladhara) without both right and left sided energies being equally balanced.

Ida	Pingala
Right cerebral hemisphere calm, relaxed state higher mental processes left nostril breath activated by oxygen slower heartbeat and respiration blue, dark, cool, negative feminine parasympathetic Yin energy	Left cerebral hemisphere, excited state, strong emotions, rational thought, physical activity, right nostril breath, activated by carbon dioxide, faster heartbeat and respiration, red, hot, positive, masculine, sympathetic, Yang energy

Applying Magnets to the Chakras

Yoga teaches that Prana is distributed throughout the body-mind through the seven chakras. Each chakra corresponds to the endocrine glands which secrete vital hormones that regulate physical activity. All the chakras are aligned along the vertical spinal column except Ajna chakra, which is located on the center of the forehead. This corresponds to the pineal gland. Sahasrara, or the crown chakra at the top of the head, corresponds to the pituitary gland.

To open chakra activity, slowly pass a bipolar U-shaped magnet of no less than 1000 gauss, but preferably higher, up the from the base of the coccyx of the spine to the top of the head, seven times in succession. Repeat this twice daily.

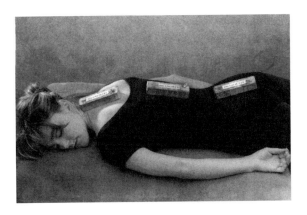

Another method is to place three South pole magnets over three important chakras such as the swadisthana or solar plexus chakra, manipura or digestive chakra, and vishuddha, thyroid or throat chakra. These will tend to open the sushumna, or Chinese Governor channel. At the same time place the Yin North pole magnet over the forehead (The head and brain usually require cooling, Yin, North pole energy). These can be applied once or twice daily for 20 to 30 minutes each time.

Muladhara

Muladhara is at the base of the spine, the center for kundalini or primal energy. In its gross form it corresponds to sexual energy.

For disorders of the reproductive system, apply the appropriate magnet to the perineum. The South pole should be applied to tone up the reproductive system, treat sterility, impotence and amenorrhea. This corresponds in TCM to Governor 1 and Conception Vessel 1, located at the perineum.

Swadisthana Chakra

The next chakra upwards from the base of the spine is roughly located between and alongside the 2nd and 3rd lumbar vertebrae and also encompasses the sacrum. This is also called the sacral plexus chakra and corresponds to the adrenals; it governs the urinary system including the kidneys, ureters and bladder. It roughly corresponds to Governor 2 and 3 and Conception Vessel 3 and 2 on the abdomen.

The North pole should be applied for constipation and genito-urinary infections and the South if there is genito-urinary weakness or diarrhea. This area also governs the lower limbs, and for conditions of numbness or paralysis one should apply the South pole; for sciatica and rheumatic pains one would apply the North pole.

Manipura Chakra

The next important chakra as we go higher on the spine is the Manipura. The term 'mani' means jewels and 'pura' means city. Literally it translates as 'City of jewels', as translated by Swami Satyananda Saraswati. It is so described because it is the center for the Fire Element which governs heat and energy. Specifically, it is described as located over the region of the spine opposite the umbilicus. According to TCM, this corresponds to Governor 4, called "Ming Men" or "Life Gate Fire," and the Conception Vessel that extends from the umbilicus down to Conception Vessel 4, located about three inches below the umbilicus point (CV8).

Applying a South pole magnet over this area will stimulate digestive processes and relieve symptoms of indigestion, bloating, food sensitivities, coldness, hypoglycemia, lack of libido and low energy. The North pole magnet can be used for lower back pain, dysentery, colitis, nervousness, hypersensitivity, loose stools and hyperacidity.

Anahata Chakra

The fourth chakra further up the spine is called Anahata chakra. It corresponds to the thymus (which is located immediately behind and slightly to the left of the breast bone or sternum), the Heart and the Lungs. It also influences the vagus nerve, which is the longest nerve in the body and enervates organic processes throughout the abdomen. Anahata chakra is aligned with the spine immediately opposite the location of the Heart. It would correspond to the territory that extends from the first to the seventh thoracic vertebrae, including acupoints Bladder 15, 14 and 13 and Governor 11 and 12 on the spine and Conception Vessel 17 on the sternum between the breasts.

The South pole is applied for cardiac weakness, low blood pressure, asthma and the later stages of pneumonia and tuberculosis.

The North pole is used for high blood pressure, palpitations, bronchitis and the earlier stages of pulmonary inflammation.

Anahata also influences the Stomach, and the North is used for ulcers, gastritis and acid eructations, while the South is used for anorexia and to stimulate appetite.

Vishuddha Chakra

Vishuddha or throat chakra is situated between the 7th cervical and 1st thoracic, also known as the brachial plexus. It specifically encompasses the parathyroid and thyroid glands and governs the eyes, ears, nose and throat. It can be considered for individuals who have difficulty expressing themselves in speech. It corresponds to Governor 14 between the 7th cervical and 1st thoracic of the spine and Conception Vessel 22 at the base of the throat.

The South pole can be used for paralytic conditions of the arms, face and low thyroid symptoms.

The North pole is indicated for stimulating the defensive system of the body, preventing and treating colds and influenza, shoulder and neck stiffness, hyperthyroidism, muscular pains of the shoulder and back.

Ajna Chakra

Ajna chakra is located in between the eyebrows or the 'third-eye' and is at the center of the brain. In Chinese medicine it is an extra point called 'Yintang'. It corresponds to the pineal gland and is the point where Ida and Pingala nadis (channels) converge. This point is sometimes regarded as the center of inner knowing or intuition. It governs the lower brain, the eyes, ears and nose. It corresponds to Yintang, located on the forehead between the eyebrows, and Governor 16 on the spine at the base of the occiput.

The South pole will stimulate mental activity while the North pole will benefit sleep, quiet the mind, aid in mental clarity and reduce epileptic seizures. It also can be used to treat migraine headaches and retarded children.

Sahasrara

The Sahasrara or crown chakra is related to the pituitary gland and externalizes at the vertex of the scalp. It corresponds to Governor 20. In Yoga, this is the place where the mystical union of Shiva (consciousness) and Shakti (energy) combine to create enlightenment. The pituitary is called the 'master gland' because it controls the entire endocrine system.

Applying the South pole at this point will stimulate mental activity and physiological processes governed by the brain throughout the body. The North pole will calm mental agitation and relieve depression.

Summary of Locations

Some authorities precisely locate the seven chakras along the front of the body as follows:

Muladhara—at the perineum, Swadisthana—the pubic bone

Manipura—the navel, Anahata—the praecordial region (heart)

Vishuddha—the base of the throat, Ajna—between the eyebrows

Treatment

Use approximately an 1100 Gauss magnet. Lay a flannel cloth over the spine of the back and position three magnets, using North pole for sedating and dispersing and South pole for tonification, corresponding to Vishuddha, Manipura and Swadisthana chakras respectively. One treatment session consists of approximately 15 to 30 minutes and the sessions can be taken twice daily.

THE USE OF NORTH AND SOUTH FACING MAGNETS ACCORDING TO JAPANESE ACUPUNCTURE PRACTICE

Most magnet therapists, including the work described in this book emphasize almost exclusively the use of the North facing magnet for most conditions. This is especially true of pain and inflammatory conditions for which magnets are particularly useful. The Japanese have used magnet therapy extensively for decades and some of the most famous therapists of the 20th century have evolved a rational and effective approach to the use of combined North and sough facing magnets. The principles of combined North and South magnets is described on page 175 of Extraordinary Vessels by Kiiko Matsumoto and Steven Birch. In general, they use 3000 gauss magnets but some have had good results with as low as 600 gauss strength.

The principles set forth by Tsugio Nagatoma and Dr. Yoshio Manaka as well as Mr. Ito are as follows:

"1. Treat the reactive area directly with the (N) 3000 and a point reflecting that area with the (S) 3000.

2. Treat the reactive area according to a left-right balance.

3. Treat the reactive area with the (N) 3000 and use the (S) 3000 further downstream on the same meridian to drain the reactive area."

The first principle suggests that one use a north magnet directly over the painful trigger point area and a south magnet over a related point according to the energetic concepts of acupuncture. For instance, if one were treating colitis or any inflammation or pain associated with the lower intestines, we would place one or more north magnets directly over the pinnacle(s) of pain on the abdomen. At the same time, since the condition involves the Large Intestine and perhaps the Stomach meridians, we would apply a north magnet on Large intestine 4 (located on the back of the hand in the space between the thumb and index finger metacarpal bones), to disperse this meridian and a south magnet on Stomach 36 (located 3 thumb widths below the lower outside edge of the knee cap, 1 thumb width outside of the mid-line of the tibia), to help draw the energy downward.

The second principle means that if one applies for instance a north magnet on the top of the wrist for carpal tunnel pain, then a south magnet would be applied on the underside. Another possibility is might be to apply a north magnet over the painful

The third principle which I have personally found to work very well is to apply a north magnet over the site of pain or inflammation and south magnets further down and above on the same approximate meridian pathway.

FURTHER CONSIDERATIONS OF HOW MAGNETS WORK

In the previous pages (page 17), a number of possible explanations have been given for why and how magnets can achieve seeming miraculous relief of pain and inflammation. After years of professional clinical use, I have a few conjectures that may prove of value.

Essentially magnets work by somehow freeing circulation of blood and bio-electrical nerve force. It is precisely the impairment of circulation that encourages the production of free radicals locally and throughout the body. Many have heard of free radicals, their harmful effects and association with degenerative disease and the need for antioxidants to counteract them. Free radicals are created as a natural by-product of everyday metabolism. Even following a healthy lifestyle and eating the most optimal diet will not completely prevent them from being created. This is why we need to eat a generous amount of vegetables, fruits, spices and herbs because these are particularly rich in polyphenols and bioflavonoids that have powerful protective effects against the ravages of free radicals.

So what is a free radical? Just as fire needs oxygen to burn, the effects of burning food for energy, environmental pollution and stress all involve the burning of oxygen. Since in its more stable form, oxygen molecules come in pairs, whenever food is metabolized or we are exposed to stress, stable oxygen molecules split forming what are known as free radicals. Each of these split oxygen molecules are compelled to further steal other molecules from various tissues resulting in a wide variety of damaging effects including inflammation, pain, accelerated aging, depressed immune system, heart diseases, arthritis and even cancer.

It seems clear that one of the mechanisms for how magnets are mechanically and safely able to achieve their phenomenal therapeutic results is that they are able to control and neutralize the pain and inflammation associated with the accumulation of free radicals at specific sites of pain and inflammation. In fact, using magnets with healthful diet and herbs is probably the best way to treat diseases caused by free radical damage to the body – which is just about all diseases.

Important New Method for Determining the Best Application of Bio-North or Bio-South Polarities

When people come to my clinic with an acute pain I have seen cases that better respond to either the north or south magnetic polarity. Thus far, my opinion is that the south polarity may be more effective for a more chronic condition while the north polarity is for more acute. However, it is not always easy to determine what the body considers a chronic or an acute reaction to be. The old method was to apply a magnet and wait for a couple of hours to a day or two to determine whether there is any benefit or if indeed one has the wrong polarity, whether the pain is the same or even a little worse. Clinically, this took time and while the north polarity works in approximately 85% of all cases of acute pain and inflammation, there are occasions when the south polarity is the effective side. Determining this, therefore, may take several days to a week.

An immediate method I have developed in my clinical practice takes less than a couple of minutes. Identify, through manual pressure, the most active trigger point associated with the patient's acute pain. This may take a little doing and there may be more than one point. Begin by applying a north-facing magnet to the trigger point and simply tap on it with the tip of your finger using medium pressure from 30 to 50 times. Then, leaving the magnet fastened to the skin with bandage tape, ask the patient to physically challenge the painful area, actually 'try to make it hurt,' of course without injuring themselves. If you have the correct polarity the pain will be significantly and noticeably relieved immediately, usually in no longer than a couple of minutes. If it is not relieved or worse, switch the magnet to the south polarity and repeat the process.

Sounds like 'strange magic'? Well, it is and it works – and like all seeming magical phenomena there will undoubtedly be discovered a physiological reason why it works. In the meantime, all magnet therapists should adopt this simple empirical clinical method.

Current Research

As yet research on the therapeutic effects of magnets are few and far between. This is because industry has not been able to determine how to profit from them. The Natural Institute of Health is rumored to have an interest in conducting research on magnet therapy. This, from an independent, non-industry aligned organization is greatly desired. However, there have been a few independent studies from respected medical doctors that have been published.

The first is an informal study by Carlos Vallbona, M.D., published in the November, 1997 issue of the Archives of Physical Medicine and Rehabilitation. The study, although very limited, involved 50 patients who were told to apply low gauss "concentric circles" type of magnets over their site of pain for only 45 minutes. After only 45 minutes, 75% reported significant pain reduction with only 19% of the patients in the control group experiencing only a slight decrease of pain.

The second is a more well designed study reported January, 1999 in the New York Times and published in the respected American Journal of Pain Management. In July, 1997, Dr. Weintraub, a clinical professor of neurology at New York Medical College, reported in a double blind study with 24 diabetic and non-diabetic patients over a period of 4 months that nine out of 10 diabetic patients reported a significant lessening of pain and 3 out of 9 patients with non-diabetic foot pain also reported significant lessening of pain.

ENDNOTES

[1] Gauss, as the measure of strength described throughout this and all other books on magnetic therapy, is very misleading, since there exists no simple standard for measuring the strength of a magnet. The strength of a magnet is determined both by its size and the material of which it is made. To date, there is no reliable measure of magnetic strength based on size and material used. Therefore, all references to so called gauss measurement used throughout this or any other book should be understood as only relative according to the size and material used.

[2] Nakagawa, Kyoichi, MD. "Magnetic Field Deficiency Syndrome & Magnetic Treatment", Japan Medical Journal, #2745, 12/4/76

[3] Morgan, Toya "Therapeutic Magnetism, Yesterday and Today" 4137 Chapman Way, Pleasanton, CA 94566, 1988 p.9

[4] Philpott, "Cancer: The Magnetic/Oxygen Answer" Philpott Medical Services, 17171 SE 29th St., Choctaw, Ok. 73020, (405) 390-3009, fax (405) 390-2968.

[5] It is interesting to compare this to tonification and sedation needle technique used by acupuncturists, where rotating a needle clockwise is tonifying while the opposite counterclockwise rotation is sedating. Similarly, shiatsu and acupressure also corroborates the opposite therapeutic significance of clockwise and counterclockwise rotation.

[6] Because of this, it is easy to disarrange the electron structure of a recording tape, CD or hard drive and thereby damage or destroy its stored information. The watchword of our high tech computer and information era is to absolutely keep all magnets away from these systems.

[7] Barefoot, Robert R. and Reich, Carl M., MD, The Calcium Factor: The Scientific Secret of Health and Youth, 1992

BIBLIOGRAPHY

Magnet Therapy Theory and Practice by Dr. Neville S. Bengali, published by Jain publishers in India, 1921, Chuna Mandi Street 10, Paharganj, New Delhi-110055

This is a very authoritative and informative book, but the reader should be aware of a semantic difference that causes the author to reverse the description of the qualities of North and South poles.

Discovery of Magnetic Health by George J. Washnis and Richard Z. Hricak, published by Nova, Rockville, Maryland, USA

Magnet Therapy by Holger Hannemann, published by Sterling publishing company, New York.

Healing Magnetism by Heinz Schiegl,. published by Weiser, York Beach, Maine

Biomagnetic Handbook by W. Philpott, MD and Sharon Taplin. Published by Enviro-Tech Products, 17171 SE 29 St., Choctaw, OK 73020. 405/390-3499

The Art of Magnetic Healing by Santwani. Published in India by Jain in New Delhi.

Magnetic Field Therapy Handbook by R. Allen Walls. Published by inner Search foundation, Inc., McLean, Virginia.

Becker, R.O. and Seldon, G. The Body Electric. Electro-Magnetism and the Foundation of Life, William Morrow & Co. New York, 1986

Becker, R.O. Cross Currents, Jeremy P. Tarcher, Inc., Los Angeles, CA 1990

SOURCES FOR MAGNETS, HERBS, BOOKS, COURSES OF STUDY & OTHER RELATED MATTERS

East West School of Herbalism
Box 712
Santa Cruz, Ca. 95061
800-717-5010   fax 408-336-3227
email: ewcourse@planetherbs.com
Offering the East West Herbal Correspondence Course and seminars by Dr. Michael Tierra and his wife, Lesley Tierra. This is a comprehensive 36 lesson course of study that integrates Western, Ayurvedic and Chinese Medicine as well as dietary and traditional diagnostic methods. Write for a complete catalogue of magnets, magnet supplies and distributor information. www.planetherbs.com

Internatural
33719 116th St-BMT
Twin Lakes, WI 53181
800-643-4221 (orders)   fax 800-905-6887
Retail supplier of herbs, books, essential oils, magnets, crystals, supplements and other alternative health and lifestyle products.

Lotus Light
PO Box 1008-BMT,
Silver Lake, WI 53170
Ph. 800-548-3824   fax 800-905-6887
Wholesale supplier of herbs, books, essential oils, magnets, crystals, supplements and other alternative health and lifestyle products.

Norso Biomagnetics
4105 Starboard CT
Raleigh, NC 27613
ph. 800-480-8601, 919-783-5911 fax 919-781-8374
They carry magnetic pads, wraps, Norso SD and Mega mattress pads, plus the special patented magnets "Magnepods" which are designed to move with the body.

Planetherbs.com
On-Line source for Magnets, Planetary Herb Formulas, Natural products at discounted prices, Books, East-West Correspondence Course, Free Forum, Articles, Chatroom and more. Its all at www.planetherbs.com.

OTHER SOURCES

AZ Industries, PO Box 250, Ash Flat, Ark. 72513, 1-501-856-3041 or fax 1-501-856-3590 This company manufactures industrial strength magnets and magnetic bars of various sizes. They will not offer any information on therapeutic use but they will send a catalogue upon request.

Health Industries Inc., Route 3, Box 121, Murray, Ky, 42071. Phone (502) 753-2613 or 1-800-626-3386.
Representing the books, products and work of Drs. Richard and Mary Broeringmeyer in the field of magnetic therapy.

Internet: A monthly Magnetic Therapy Research Bulletin: WWW.Buhyl.com

Magna-Pak Inc. PO Box 27106, London, Ontario, Canada, N5X 3X5 USA office 3560 Pine Grove #315, Port Huron, Mi. 48060
1-800-361-1387; Fax 519-660-8386
Internet: Http://www.lonet.ca/comm/Magna-Pak
Website: www.magnapak.com

Mid-American Marketing - Magnetic Specialities and More
1531 E. Main Street
Eaton, Ohio 45320
1-800-922-1744; 937-456-9393
Fax: 937-456-9897
E-Mail: maml@infinet.com

Naturheilpraxis
Post Box 149
Ch-9101 Herisau
Switzerland
This company distributes various types of therapeutic magnets including magnet foils.

Oriental Medical Supply, 1950 Washington St., Braintree, Mass. 02184, USA, phone 1-800-323-1839 or fax 1 617-335-5779
They have a wide range of all the different kinds and forms of magnets discussed in this article.

Philpott Medical Services, 17171 Se. 29th St., Choctaw, OK., 73020, Phone (405) 390-3009, Fax (405) 390-2968
They have a variety of highly authoritative books on magnetic therapies and products.

PsychoPhysics Labs, 4264 Topsail Ct., Soquel, CA 95073. Manufactures pulsed magnetic generators and other instruments.

Relaxus Massage Products, 4550 Birch Bay/Lynden Rd., Blaine, Washington 98230
1-800-668-9876, fax 1-604-879-0889
Head Office 2020 Manitoba Court, Vancouver, BC V5Y 3V3
Schafer's Health Centre LTD, Box 251, Unity, Sask., Canada S0K 4L0
Telephone 1 306-228-2512

Space Age Bio-magnetic Products 27134A Paseo Espada, Ste. 303, San Juan Capistrano, CA 92675. Tel (949) 248-5212, Fax (949) 248-5212, 1-800-861-0513
Website: Http://www.spaceage.com
E-Mail: spaceage@spaceage.com
They have a wide variety of biomagnetic products, including unique jewelry items, face masks and home magnetic water softeners.

PLANETARY HERBOLOGY

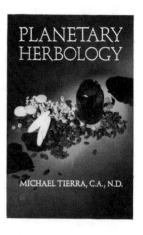

Michael Tierra, C.A., N.D.

$17.95; 485 pp.;
5½ × 8½ paper; charts.
ISBN: 0941-524272

Lotus Press is pleased to announce a new practical handbook and reference guide to the healing herbs, a landmark publication in this field. For unprecedented usefulness in practical applications, the author provides a comprehensive listing of the more than 400 medicinal herbs available in the west. They are classified according to their chemical constituents, properties and actions, indicated uses and suggested dosages. Students of eastern medical theory will find the western herbs cross-referenced to the Chinese and Ayurvedic (Indic) systems of herbal therapies. This is a useful handbook for practitioners as well as readers with a general interest in herbology.

Michael Tierra, C.A., N.D., whose very popular earlier book, *THE WAY OF HERBS,* led the way to this new major work. He is one of this country's most respected herbalists, a practitioner and teacher who has taught and lectured widely. His eclectic background studies in American Indian herbalism, the herbal system of Dr. John Christopher, and traditional oriental systems of India and China, contributes a special richness to his writing.

To order your copy, send $19.95 (postpaid) to:
Lotus Press
P.O. Box 325-BMT
Twin Lakes, WI 53181
Request our complete book & sidelines catalog.
Wholesale inquiries welcome.